HAIR L(

HAIR LOSS AND WIGS
A woman's dilemma and how to win through

Ruth Lewis-Browning

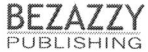
BEZAZZY
PUBLISHING

Published by Bezazzy Publishing
www.bezazzypublishing.co.uk

ISBN 0 9550667 1 9

British Library Cataloguing in Publication Data.
A catalogue record for this book is available from the British Library.

Designed and typeset by Bezazzy Publishing
Cover design © Bzp 2005

Printed and bound in Great Britain
by Antony Rowe Ltd, Eastbourne

CONTENTS

Introduction

Everyone loses hundreds of hairs from their head every day. It's a natural and regenerative process and more hair is growing at the same time. Yet sometimes more is lost than is being replaced so that thin patches start to appear. Losing one's hair is nearly always a concern, at whatever age, and however partial or temporary it might turn out to be. It can be particularly difficult for a woman, since fundamentally it represents a loss of an important aspect of femininity.

Hair loss may develop in many situations, perhaps the two best known being stress-related alopecia and as a side effect of chemotherapy. In both instances, hair growth is expected to resume in time. However, sometimes it does not, especially where the loss has resulted from a traumatic event not associated transparently with physical illness. Sometimes too an injury leaves scars over which hair will not be able to return, or there is a family tendency towards thinning hair. The condition of hair loss can be extensive and lifelong and it may also affect all parts of the body including, more noticeably, the eyelashes and eyebrows.

When we meet such a difficulty, naturally we turn to the medical professions to help us, reassured that someone will be able to make the diagnosis and that the right cure can be prescribed or administered. It is only when experiencing the condition first hand that one realises this is an area in which medical science cannot yet provide all the answers for everyone.

Any search of publications or the Internet will return lists of studies of types of hair loss, academic or self-help papers assigning names to the various degrees of loss, and books explaining theories about why it occurs. There are drawings that illustrate graphically one condition or another, as well as copious sources of suggested remedies, drugs and treatments, some potentially more effective or suitable than others. Magazines or television programmes may from time to time relate the story of a particular sufferer, often someone new to the condition, who feels that their life has been devastated. Yet very little guidance is available to assist the embarrassed or distressed sufferer to manage on a very practical and day-to-day basis.

What is it really like for a woman to lose her hair and what are all the new difficulties that have to be faced? Quite simply what do you do about it? Is it possible to go swimming? Can a wig be washed? How do you cope with wearing a wig for the first time on a windy day.... and for longer? What types of wig are available and where can you get one? I have written this book as a real and genuine hair loss sufferer who unexpectedly lost all hair in adulthood and is facing up to a life long condition. I have tried just about every trick of the 'trade' to find the best way of adapting to hair loss and to buying and wearing full wigs for many work, domestic and social situations.

This is the book that every female hair loss sufferer should read because I look at real life issues from an entirely non-medical perspective, from handling the sensitivities of relationships to coping effectively with the discomfort of wearing a wig during hot weather. My aim is to give other hair loss sufferers some really helpful hints and tips for dealing with the problem in a practical and positive way. I hope that the book will also prove useful to those who give care and support to hair loss sufferers and that it will become an aid to much greater and general understanding.

Ruth Lewis-Browning
2005

1

Finding there's a problem

Time stops for a moment and it feels like the end of normality. Anyone who has seen the first hair on the pillow in the morning, or felt a small patch of scalp where hair really should be, will recognise that moment of realisation. There may be an extra few hairs lingering in the bathroom basin after shampooing, or the hairbrush may seem to be gathering rather more bits than usual. It's barely noticeable at first, but then the awful truth begins to dawn. Hair is starting to fall out. Surely, this can't really be happening?

Let no one ever underestimate what it feels like to a woman to know that she may be losing her hair. It doesn't matter whether it is just a small amount or if it is only supposed to be temporary. It doesn't even matter if she knows in advance that it is going to happen, maybe because of a particular medical treatment, and so she has had time to prepare herself. Seeing the first hairs falling out is simply the worst kind of moment.

Feminine hair loss can be horrifying and upsetting. Yet why should anyone feel like this? Why is it so momentous to a woman when she starts to lose her hair and how can she cope with the visible and social effects of the hair loss?

Why hair is important

In many cultures, a woman's hair is considered to be her crowning glory, even though she may often complain about it! It's what makes her look the way she is, it is often admired and it's what she dresses when she goes out. She may use a new style to make her feel good at an occasion, or she may want to look attractive to a prospective or current partner. One only needs to take a look at all the commercial hair products on the market to know how important it all is. The shops are filled with rows and rows of lotions and potions purporting to clean, condition, straighten, curl or colour.

There are training courses and examinations for hair stylists, innovative salon equipment and hair products, hair massage and pampering treatments, specialist salon interior designers, even international competitions and awards for hair cuts and creations. Just about every modern city, town and village has its street corner business with the familiar row of basins and dryers and the warm, slightly perfumed smell that wafts out of an open door on a summer day. Every woman is expected to have hair, and most to want to groom it, and an entire industry (and 'makeover' trend) has developed around this expectation. If having lovely hair makes a woman feel good, conversely having poor or no hair can make her feel dreadful.

Having head hair is an important part of the modern human being. In particular it helps to protect us from excesses of light, heat and cold. Yet in the author's view its enormous significance to modern living is often grossly underestimated. Having one's hair 'done' by a professional hairdresser is part of a restorative process, some would say an essential one, although most will not think of it in such a way. Going to the hairdresser can give the customer a very pleasant after-effect, though this is usually just associated with having a new or tidier look. However, there is probably far more to it than this. Tending the hair, or touching the head, is one of those mysterious sensual activities that if correctly carried out can make the whole of the body feel calm and correctly balanced.

Some cultures and some therapists do of course recognise that it is significantly beneficial and relaxing to feel trained human hands on any part of the head, especially if the scalp is massaged carefully. This may also be part of a programme of washing with perfumed lotions. However, when the hair is no longer there to be washed and tended, an important part of the physical body's opportunity for reaching a state of well-being has been removed. Thus too, an important part of physical therapy can no longer be applied and enjoyed, unless of course the hair loss sufferer is prepared to expose the often embarrassing condition to others, perhaps to a scalp massage therapist, or to purchase an item of head massage-delivering equipment. Washing one's own hair or massaging one's own head induces a good sensation, but this is never as good as relaxing whilst someone else does the work.

Having head hair can be immensely enjoyable, as well as a bit of a practical nuisance. It gives us many of life's pleasures. A baby or small child will reach out and make contact with a mother's hair. A woman's hair can play an important tactile part in adult relationships, making its imperfection or loss a great contributor to difficulties between some partners. Those who do not have a partner may find the prospect of starting new relationships becomes a daunting and prohibitive one, because inevitably hair loss has to be revealed or explained.

What hair loss means to a woman

Most significantly of all, head hair is a fundamental part of being feminine. It is one of a range of important physical signals that helps to differentiate between adult male and adult female. Although there are certainly no hard and fast rules - with some women opting to wear shaven head styles and some men preferring long and luxurious tresses - in general terms only men are 'supposed' to lose their head hair involuntarily.

Inadvertently, the actions of some men can also make the problem seem more acute to a female hair loss sufferer. Men who want to express a feminine persona may sometimes try to mimic what they regard as a fundamental woman's appearance via the wearing of supplementary or full hairpieces. Head hair is what a woman is expected to have. To look like a woman, such men want to wear a good head of hair.

So the unwanted feminine loss of head hair can be particularly embarrassing, annoying, physically difficult and even mentally devastating. Furthermore, in whatever circumstances it might occur, it is almost always a previously unexpected event in a woman's life. Although some young people may (more rarely) experience hair loss conditions, including the very youngest of children, it is perhaps a particular shock for a woman who has for many years enjoyed a good head of hair. She may have felt is was part of what attracted a partner to her, or she may have regarded its grooming as an essential part of her personality or career image.

Hair loss can cause many tears, depression, deep sadness, and even desperation. It can make a sufferer want to crawl away and avoid being seen. It can ruin lives and even tear apart relationships. It can lead to concern and anxiety of a magnitude that to others seems way beyond the visible evidence. Those feelings are real and all consuming to the woman who first faces the stark reality that her hair is falling out.

Seeking help

Even now, too little is known about some hair loss conditions, about why they happen to some people but do not happen to others and what if anything can be done to help. This fact alone makes the experience seem so much more isolating. Sometimes it seems that there is just no one to ask who can help make it all better.

But this does not mean that help should not be sought. If a woman has any hair loss whatsoever, she should always talk in the first instance to her own doctor. There may be a very simple and identifiable reason for the condition in a particular patient and, happily, an equally simple solution. It may be associated with a skin infection or period of stress. There may be a family tendency towards feminine hair loss so it will help if a patient can make known anything they might also suspect from the family history. Occasionally it may also indicate that there is some other underlying medical problem that should and could be treated successfully.

So in the first instance all female hair loss sufferers should share all concerns with a medical adviser. Things may not be as bad as they seem at first and the health expert can give reassurance and help to decide on the best course of action. A medical practitioner will probably want to examine the scalp with a magnifying instrument and ask other questions about general health and lifestyle. A patient may be referred to a dermatologist or other specialist at a hospital.

Unfortunately, seeking help is one of the first major hurdles facing any hair loss sufferer. Precisely because it is distressing and embarrassing to lose one's hair, making the evidence of this known to anyone else, even a trusted doctor, can be an extremely difficult thing for some people.

You are not on your own

If you are reading this because you are a female sufferer of hair loss, then be assured that I know exactly what you may be feeling. I have shed so many tears since the problems first started. It all began around the time of my pregnancies. During my first, I developed pre-eclampsia, another condition of women for which effective treatments still seem woefully in short supply. My illness all but led to my own fatality and alas did lead to our daughter's stillbirth, her death occurring traumatically three days before her natural delivery. Being the baby's mother and thus 'responsible' for her during her development, it was impossible to avoid recurring feelings of intense guilt. The sense of deep loss was indescribable. A comment that perhaps I could consider acquiring a puppy or a kitten instead, though undoubtedly a very kindly and well-meant suggestion, did in fact feel like one of the most upsetting at that time.

According to the 'textbooks', I was expected to recover from the eclamptic condition very quickly after the delivery. In fact soon after returning home I became steadily worse and was rushed back to hospital, with swollen limbs, a severe headache and my eyes seeing the world only in shades of navy blue. Happily, I did recover physically, although it took many weeks. The emotional scars have been much harder to manage. Then, two further pregnancies ended in late miscarriages and my chances of having a family faded away, the upset compounded by incoming junk mail targeted at smiling pregnant mothers and relating to adorable baby clothes and financial investments for the new family. Our waiting 'nursery' became the 'spare room' and then, to my final and utter dismay, my hair began to fall out.

Eventually I returned to work and soon I had to wear a wig to cover up the expanding and thinning patches. When my colleagues commented favourably on my new hairstyle, I made poor excuses and never admitted that I was wearing a wig. Of course they probably realised that I was, but they were polite enough to gloss over it. It would have been so much better if I had felt able to be more open about the whole thing. If any one of those colleagues had actually asked me directly if I was wearing a wig, I would probably have been relieved and would have replied 'yes' and 'please help'. I just didn't have the courage to open the subject myself first.

My type of work meant that I was visible to all kinds of people throughout the day and occasionally I even had to work in front of cameras. It was a time of great worry about how I looked and my confidence was eroding quickly. I began to feel physically sick during the morning drives to work, sometimes having to stop the car for a while, and I came to dread going to a job that I had once been so keen to secure. A little later, when an opportunity came to do something completely different, I was greatly relieved to call it a day. At times like this, one needs either a vast amount of proactive support, or to make a break for it and have a fresh start where questions may not have to be answered.

It was not long before all my hair had gone. I have not had any hair for more than a decade since then, not only on my head but progressively just about everywhere else including eyelashes and eyebrows. Even seeing my old makeup bag could reduce me to floods of tears. It seemed a double blow to go through all the trauma, have none of the hoped-for children, and only be left with an embarrassing hair loss problem.

It is natural to place the blame for all this on the extremes that I went through both physically and mentally. I wondered too if there could be some direct link between hair loss and the condition of pre-eclampsia that has yet to be identified? Perhaps my hair would have fallen out anyway, without the trauma or the pregnancies, due to some pre-programmed genetic blueprint? It seems that for the time being at least no one can be sure. But the outcome was without doubt. My hair was falling out, little by little, and then more and more, until one day it had all disappeared.

Whatever the circumstances and reason for anyone's hair loss, the daily hurdles may be the same. It is not intended here to be simply an outpouring of emotion, although perhaps I may be forgiven for including some of these 'hurts' along the way. Anyone reading this because they have their own hair loss has been through or is now experiencing many of their own personal difficulties. I don't really need to tell them anything more in this respect, but I do hope that having read about a few of my experiences they may take comfort that there are many more of us out there.

There are also numerous help and support groups where a sufferer can meet with others undergoing the same or similar difficulties, can share experiences and tips, even make new friends and learn to laugh about things. I did not join any such group, simply because I am naturally a shy and private person who dislikes large social and group occasions. But I know that these can be immensely helpful to many and should be recommended. If you are interested, ask at your local medical surgery or hospital department if you are not sure where to find points of contact. Most of all, do not be afraid to go along to meet others for the first time. Everyone there will be in the same boat and will be exceedingly understanding and sympathetic. They really want and need you to join them, especially so that the numbers of people in their own situation can grow and a local shared self-help network can be strengthened and expanded.

If there are no help groups available in your area, you may be the kind of person who could consider establishing one. That way, any adverse feelings about your own misfortune can be channelled positively into helping others. You may be able to foster the support of a local radio station or newspaper. There are always opportunities to give talks at meetings or as part of training courses, at women's groups and healthcare events. Although the subject seems very specific, practical knowledge about hair loss, its impact and consequences, can be extremely useful as part of a wide range of medical, therapy, psychology, counselling, community, social education and training courses.

You may find it helpful to write down how you feel, expressing your concerns in a way that is not so easy verbally. Pass your notes to a medical practitioner or carer and invite them to be used in the training of other professionals. You have valuable experience to share that is not included in most of their textbooks.

Sharing the experience

This is not the place to discuss in detail the various medical conditions and treatments associated with hair loss, for of course there are those who are far better qualified and there is plenty of literature on these elsewhere. Rather I shall now be moving on to do some straight talking purely from the sufferer's point of view, looking at day-to-day obstacles from my own direct experience and suggesting effective ways to overcome them, so that those with hair loss can start to regain their confidence and turn an apparent difficulty into something much more constructive.

Unfortunately, many who suffer hair loss do have at some time or another to consider wearing a partial or full wig. I do now wear a full wig, all the time and long-term. This has been a massive psychological and practical hurdle to overcome. Only those who have to deal personally with this can really know what it feels like. It is indescribably awful to have to move from own hair to false hair. There can be few things worse to happen to a woman than losing any aspect of her femininity and appearance.

I have thought for a long time about whether or not I should write this book, since by its very content it exposes many of my own private thoughts and experiences that I have for so long been striving to conceal. On many occasions I have started and then set the project aside. But I have gone ahead because I want to try to answer for others the kinds of questions that no one could answer for me when I first started to lose my hair. It is the kind of book that I always wanted to read but could never find. Once the medical profession had gone as far as it could with me, I was left on my own to face up to the world. What on earth was I going to do and how was I going to deal with my hair loss? How was I going to get hold of a suitable wig if I needed one, how did I keep it firmly on my head and how could I ever feel able to meet people face to face again?

The chapters that follow look at the everyday realities directly from the 'patient' point of view. I shall talk particularly about situations that cause new practical difficulties, about coping with the buying and wearing of full wigs, both artificial fibre and human hair, with plenty of genuine hints and tips. Much of what I have to say may be of especial interest to the longer-term wig wearers.

Alongside this, I hope that those who are supporting hair loss sufferers - be they medical staff, carers, family or friends - may be able to gain a greater understanding of what hair loss is really like to the sufferer on a daily basis and what practical things they can suggest that will be well received and that really do help.

Although much of what I have already said about my own past experiences may seem critical of some sections of the health care services, this is of course only based on one circumstance and may not be very typical. Indeed I owe a very great personal debt to some and am in great admiration of numerous others. There are many who are highly dedicated, caring and skilled, and who will always endeavour to go out of their way to find out what it is like at the patient's end of the process, so that they will be better equipped to help future patients who have sensitive problems such as hair loss. This is another reason why I have decided to publish about this most difficult of subjects.

I shall never pretend that everything can be solved, or that the difficulty can be made to go away. However, there are many things that my husband and I have learnt along the way as we have dealt with our own experiences and now I want to pass this knowledge on to others.

2

Little things

L ike any adverse condition in life, the first stages to recovery are recognising, accepting and then understanding the problem. But if anyone tries to find any woman with the first stages of hair loss who wants either to admit it to herself or to make it known to others, then they will most probably be unsuccessful. 'Absolutely not', will be her likely response. The most natural reaction of all is to want to cover it up, hoping it will get better and that in the meantime nobody will notice. And that is exactly what almost every woman will do.

What is often overlooked is that hair loss is also a most difficult condition for the sufferer's family or friends to approach. This is because in the early stages the physical effects are probably still being kept from their view. It is rather like the amount of sympathy normally given to an apparent back pain sufferer, as opposed to that lavished on someone with a scar or perhaps a leg in plaster. It is so much easier to understand and deal with the blatantly visible.

Unfortunately, in trying to be helpful to a hair loss sufferer, for instance by touching the hair to help cover up any exposed tell tale patches (especially at the back or on top of the head) this may only make them feel that the problem must thus be really obvious simply because it has been noticed. The sensitivity with which many women regard hair loss can be absolutely monumental.

First realisations

When the little thin patches first started to appear on my head they would come and go at different places. I was told that the 'alopecia' would get better as I recovered from my bad experiences associated with the pregnancies. It was just a matter of time. This did not make me feel any better about it or help the problem to go away. It was purely and simply just devastating. I waited and hoped. But it got worse until all hair had gone. More than ten years later I am still waiting and hoping for it to return.

At first I tried the comb-over approach to disguise the difficulty, covering thin patches with adjacent hair, then also using hair lacquer to keep the coverage firmly in place over the thin areas. This was reasonably successful at first, but I did not really like using hairsprays, especially if strongly-perfumed, and it was difficult to apply enough to the offending points without creating a flat, sticky patch that might draw attention anyway. It meant constant monitoring in two small mirrors, diving into rest room cubicles when out and about, and fiddling to get a view of the right part of my head whilst making any adjustments.

The added dilemma now was whether or not I should still be able go to a hairdresser. A 'clever cut' can cover up a lot of the problem in the early or temporary stages. But how could I depend on a stylist not to let the problem show during cutting and not to mention it within earshot of others. Would the salon keep me protected from the curious eyes of other customers? Hairdressing salons can be very public places at the best of times, often with broad shop windows to the street outside, and of course all the staff and many of the customers have a fantastic view of the top and back of one's head. Then having plucked up courage and gained the sympathetic ear of one trusted stylist, another unaware junior might be asked to do the shampooing. The joy of having someone pamper my hair, something I had always loved and had taken for granted, was now becoming a potential nightmare. I started to grow my hair into something longer that probably I could deal with myself.

The next trick was to adopt a style with which I could try to disguise patches, by tying hair back and pinning it in place, by using a hair band, slides or fancy clips. These were quite fashionable at the time, though really a little too young-looking as I entered my middle age. It did make me feel a little more 'secure' though and meant that I could use something sparkly for an evening out. I began to hate anyone standing behind me, always feeling that they were staring at my hair, and I wanted to avoid sitting in theatres or rooms where there were others likely to be positioned immediately behind. As I am not a tall person and others often look physically downwards to me, this seemed to make worse the feeling of observation.

The simple opening of the house door to a known mail deliverer also now required more consideration. I had to make doubly sure that everything hair-wise was in its proper place before I 'emerged'. A mirror in the hall became essential. Attending to an occasional early morning delivery from a courier was another new concern, especially when I needed to put on a wig first and check that it was brushed into a reasonable shape.

Considering treatments

There are products on the market which can be used to apply colour to bare parts of the scalp and for many this helps to disguise a small or temporary problem. Where there is a reasonable amount of hair either side of a thin patch, a coloured volumising spray or foam can be very helpful and effective. But many of us just do not like to keep spraying chemicals and potions on our hair, so this is only a suitable route for some sufferers, and again it requires time for some advance work before feeling ready to meet people. The subject of surgical hair transplantation has always sounded far too horrific to me and like any surgical procedure there are bound to be all sorts of discomforts and risk factors. One thing is probably certain. Concealing evidence of the problem is definitely not an option during such kinds of treatment.

The final medical treatment I underwent was to receive intense light to try to re-stimulate head hair growth. For this I was classed as a Dermatology patient. The light was administered under strictly controlled conditions at hospital and involved first having my head covered with a sensitising lotion. Then, with the rest of my body protected, I stood upright inside a narrow and temporarily sealed cubicle, which issued hot light like an upright sun bed. As I have a tendency towards claustrophobia and also at the time was coping with particularly uncomfortable menopausal hot flushes (also called 'hot flashes'), this treatment became a considerable ordeal and caused me much private distress. Furthermore, the lotion was always applied by a different set of duty staff, each of whom asked me the same questions about my condition which I had already found embarrassing to have to answer once. Then, due to the physical layout of the department, I was also obliged to walk to the light treatment cubicle across a corridor that held other patients waiting for different treatments, causing me further acute embarrassment.

After a few weeks, a member of the hospital staff suggested to me that my hair loss was not showing any signs of recovery and that I might think about whether I wished to continue with this particular treatment. On this basis, I did not. So I was very unhappy to hear much later of the apparent report that I was not actually co-operating with this treatment. I had always taken the view that I would do anything at all that might help and I would certainly have been prepared to continue if the advice had been communicated differently.

I understand that some success has been achieved through the use of steroid injections to re-stimulate hair growth, although this was not offered to me. However, as far as I am aware, these are made directly into the scalp so are of course not without considerable discomfort. Some hair may grow back, but in my own view unless sufficient hair returns so that a wig does not have to be worn, then all the pain is probably without any real long-term gain. However, seeing some hair re-grow can be a great boost to confidence and in some cases a small amount of re-growth might be enough to trigger a fuller recovery of hair. This kind of treatment is perhaps most likely to be successful immediately there is a problem and whilst the hair growing system is still reasonably 'active'.

A few may benefit from the application of a lotion to induce scalp irritation, and thus stimulate re-growth, but clearly each individual must consider whether the practical difficulties of this make it worth a try. The head needs to be uncovered at times and will of course be intensely itchy or sore. A range of other medication and drugs has also been developed, with some items available at high street pharmacies or via the Internet, bringing varying levels of success depending on the nature and extent of the hair loss problem. Personally, I would urge anyone to proceed with great caution when considering a programme of medication because with all drugs there can be known or unforeseen side effects. Always discuss such things with a doctor first, and especially if you are already taking other medication.

Where hair growth fails, there are any number of artificial hair products, especially full wigs, that can disguise the difficulties highly effectively and without any physical intrusions. As a long-term wig wearer, I have accumulated considerable experience of such things and have come to know the daily hurdles that have to be faced.

Everyday obstacles

Others should understand that there are a number of normal everyday activities that will now instil anything from reluctance to terror for the embarrassed hair loss sufferer. Particularly worrying are things or actions that can displace a carefully arranged style. It is helpful if everyone associated with someone with hair loss can be aware of the main worries and always keep these in mind. I have listed some of the fears at the end of the book, but meanwhile here are a few examples:

Going to the opticians

Three particular situations come to mind in which I have found myself in situations that induce great anxiety. Firstly, a trip to the opticians. I wear spectacles and always have to put them on with a degree of care so as not to displace my wig around the top and back of the ears. Those who have had an eye test will recall the process. It often involves wearing a series of optical devices into which different lenses are slotted, as well as resting the chin, face or whole head on a number of different pieces of equipment. For the wig-wearer this simple episode can become one to dread, simply because the items used to conduct the test can dislodge hair or cause embarrassment when wig wearing has to be explained. Loss of eyelashes may also cause worry about close up tests, or may leave eyes unprotected from dust that can affect contact lens wearers.

The test is not too bad an experience when it is conducted in private and as a one-to-one session. A quiet word about one's situation is relatively easy to deal with. However, most optician businesses complete the choosing and fitting of frames in the open shop area. Putting on and taking off a number of frames is tricky for a wig-wearer, for the reasons mentioned above, but the measuring and post-delivery fitting are a great worry. These always seem to involve the practitioner or assistant fiddling about with the hair around the ear area. If you can wear 'contacts', of course this will help.

On one occasion, in a leading chain of opticians, I decided to have a precautionary word with the principal assistant in advance, expecting that she would then be able to take my concerns into account. I started to relax when as a result of our conversation she dealt with me directly for the fitting stage. However, her time to 'clock off' arrived and without a word to me she handed over to a very junior assistant who also led me to sit at another fitting point, this one in full view of the busy high street outside. It was extremely upsetting. Yet I felt unable to protest or explain to the youngster because the shop was filled with other customers. My solution has since been to find a privately owned business where the staff members have come to know me and I can attend without fear of embarrassment.

The dental visit

Another situation that used to give me concern is the routine dental inspection, although this usually causes rather less difficulty than the opticians or doctor's appointments.

There are two particular areas to think about – leaning back carefully on a reclining dentist chair (in case the wig moves or even falls off as I am moved backwards) and wearing the protective eye goggles that are mostly required (which can push a wig out of position if they are not put on with care). Some dental assistants want to be helpful by putting the goggles on for you, so this is easily dealt with by intervening and making sure you do this for yourself.

I deal with the first problem by ensuring that my head always leans firmly on the headrest of the chair, *before* the recliner begins to be lowered, and staying in that position until the chair is fully back up straight again and I can 'detach' myself and sit upright. Fortunately, my dental practice is progressive and relaxed and I have not experienced too many difficulties in this respect, feeling able to mention the problem if it seems appropriate.

Your dentist may ask routinely if you have any medical conditions or changes in health since a previous visit. It is always best to mention any hair loss problem as this may prove to be reflected in other conditions. For instance, a dermatologist pointed out pitting on my finger nails which is associated with alopecia conditions.

The medical examination

A further area of concern is the routine medical examination but especially the preventative smear test sessions that most ladies will be invited to attend at some time or another. Any loss of body hair makes this potentially and acutely embarrassing.

Fortunately, because of the nature of the test, these are usually undertaken in private cubicles by a trained nurse or other medical practitioner, who will be very understanding and certainly not in any way bothered about it. If this sort of event worries you, it is always the best policy to mention your condition to the person taking the sample before things get underway, or take a trusted family member or friend with you who can help to explain your concerns.

Never avoid a preventative test or examination just because you may be embarrassed by it. It isn't worth it. Many very serious diseases can be halted or cured if they are discovered early enough and falling ill is so very much worse than a few moments of being embarrassed.

A little understanding

The lady hair loss sufferer can become nervy and will want to shy away from many situations that others regard as perfectly normal. She will probably need to be eased through with a level of patient understanding (without knowingly drawing special attention) and careful thought (please never hand her the grasping new baby to admire without asking first!). It is a question of gradually restoring confidence and self-esteem. Much will also depend on how confident a person the sufferer was before losing hair. Every person will react in a different way and the carer needs to make a very careful assessment of the whole person, of their previous character and general lifestyle.

Some sufferers will feel able to talk about their situation quite readily, whilst others may take years before they feel able to do this. Unlike a number of other physical disabilities, hair loss can generate a sense of amusement and ridicule and those with more advanced conditions will be acutely aware of this prospect. Although most men have to accept balding as they grow older, this is not generally expected of women unless they are undergoing short term medical treatments. Alas, our current social conventions make it largely unacceptable for a woman to be seen partly or totally hairless, whereas a man with the same condition may find himself being the butt of mild shared jokes but nevertheless will not be regarded as anything unusual.

Life would be much easier in our fashion-conscious society if none of us had head hair at all, or we all shaved it off. It would certainly be a lot cheaper too! Many men would probably agree.

3

All the way

M ost people with a small amount of head hair loss, who have thin patches or are undergoing treatments such as chemotherapy, will eventually regain their hair. If you have hair loss now, you may well have hair again quite quickly. There is always that hope and for most it is a very real prospect. Every situation is different and it is one of those conditions in life that will have an unpredictable outcome. Happily, if hair decides to re-grow, its return can be astonishingly rapid and complete. Although the difficulties associated with the loss are very acute at the time, some comfort can be derived from knowing that it might not be for long. If you're 'lucky', it may simply be that a period of stress has caused the problem. Remove the stress and back come the locks.

Carers should understand that experiencing and dealing with the shock and dismay of hair loss can create its own new feelings of stress that compound the condition and also have to be addressed. Even during what turns out to be temporary loss, whilst it lasts it can be as bad to the sufferer as having permanent difficulties, precisely because no one knows exactly when things might return to normal. There is also the possibility that someone who has once experienced a period of alopecia will also experience a return of that condition, sometimes several times. Thus the regaining of confidence can be an extremely lengthy process.

Longer-term hair loss

There are those for whom hair loss does become very much more of a long-term and therefore a lifestyle changing condition. I am such a person. For me the realisation that the hair is just refusing to return was probably one of the most devastating days of my life. Despite the endless medical tests and examinations, the creams and potions, the massages and heat treatments, the positive thinking, the blasting with light and the lowering of stress, it refused to grow back as expected. Something in my hair-making mechanism has simply decided to switch off and medical science apparently cannot be sure why it has happened or what can be done about it.

Losing hair does not necessarily mean that there is any other health problem, the only other outward effect being possibly the light pitting of finger nails. Inevitably, the lack of a direct life-threatening scenario makes the problem fall further down the list of medical research priorities. Admittedly there are any number of booklets and websites that explain about types of hair loss and associated treatments, but unfortunately an equal number which see only commercial gain and quite frankly do not always give entirely correct or up to date information. If in doubt, it is always best to check with a qualified and registered medical practitioner.

The truth began to dawn on me that I was going to be pretty much on my own with hair loss, that is, just husband and me. The hair was going quickly and I now had to resort to wearing a wig in public. I hated looking in a mirror. It just did not seem to be the right sort of me any more. If I caught sight of myself in a shop window or mirror when out and about I was horrified and felt that my wig was surely obvious to everyone. However, if I had looked harder in the reflections I might have observed that actually no one around me was taking any notice at all. At such times one can become totally preoccupied with appearance and what other people are thinking. I recall a television documentary on the subject where a lady had taken to remaining in her house alone much of the time, simply because she could not come to terms with hair loss and wearing a wig in public. She was surrounded by boxes and boxes of different wigs, but couldn't bring herself to be seen in them. She was in mental torture. This should never, never have to happen.

One of the things I came to miss most was that I could not enjoy the pleasant smell of fresh shampoo on my own hair, or experience that lovely clean feeling of soft hair after a shower. Until now I had taken such things entirely for granted. I would also have to miss feeling the wind in my hair on a holiday walk, something that I had always loved so much. I had been brought up near a high moorland area and adored wild, exhilarating days on 'the top of the world'. What was I going to do?

How would I cope? I asked the inevitable question of why did it have to happen to me? Most of all, what did my husband think and would he still love me?

One copes because one has to cope. There isn't a choice (which is pretty unfair) but, well, there it all is. And a loving partner minds a whole lot less about what you look like than a hair loss sufferer thinks. They love *you*. The real you. The you that is *always* there. And if you suffer, so do they, because they don't like to see you in difficulty. Of course for their own sake and how they want to present you to friends and colleagues, they don't want your real hair to go either! They want to help, so do not exclude them. It affects you both. Bring them in on everything and work things out together. And if there is no sympathetic partner around to work with, then it is important to find a friend or counsellor who can share concerns. There is absolutely no need to handle this thing alone. My husband and I have now agreed that we are both best described as 'folically challenged', except he still needs to go to a hairdresser or barber and show feigned amusement about men who do not have quite so much 'on top' these days.

Although I am not discussing male hair loss here, I do want everyone to remember that men are sensitive too, even though they are not expected always to show it. If you have hair loss yourself, take another look at your male partner or male friends and do not concentrate exclusively on your own situation to the exclusion of the underlying personal concerns of others. Thinking about others also helps to make your own problem seem a little less all-consuming.

Talking about it

It is so much easier to say 'let's talk' about feminine hair loss than it is to go and do the actual talking. It took me many years of covering up, and then the wig wearing (more on this later), before I could talk openly about my experience. Then one day, having left my work and started a new kind of life (not as a direct result of the hair loss), I decided to be proactive and to tell people about my hair problem. My thinking was that if everyone knew, then I would no longer have to fear them finding out or noticing anything unusual.

I started with my immediate family, then neighbours and friends. The first one was scary. Then another breath-holding bit was when I had been able to tell one family relative, but had not yet got to talk to another who might communicate with the first in the mean time! This was a useful thought though, because it spurred me on to complete the task very quickly with everyone else. No turning back.

Interestingly, without exception they seemed a lot less bothered than I had anticipated they would be. It was almost deflating! After all those years struggling with one of the biggest concerns of my entire life, it did not seem to matter particularly to anyone else. Why could they not give me a bit more reaction? Why weren't they absolutely horrified? Of course, I realised that they probably knew about or suspected the problem for much longer, but they certainly had the good grace not to show this to my face. One or two seemed a little uncomfortable about what to say to me in reply on the subject, but it soon passed and they have since apparently chosen never to mention it to me again. However, the best and most important outcome was that I felt as if a great weight had been lifted.

My recommendation to any new sufferer is to cut out the secretive stage altogether if you possibly can. Go on. Just go for it. Try to overcome the seemingly tremendous hurdle of admitting the problem as early as you can, even if it is only to confide in one close friend. Once you have done it, then there is so much less to fear. It is an old cliché, but a problem shared really is a problem halved. If the hair problem lasts longer than expected, then anyway eventually you will have to deal with people knowing about it. So why not get it out of the way and over with? It is much better to get in first, before people start whispering. Then there is nothing about which they can whisper. Go for some well-deserved sympathy, for you really deserve it. Without a doubt, they will surely want some sympathy themselves for their own ailments when they arise. After all, it can be really annoying when people complain to you about their seemingly far more minor ailments, when you have been suffering your own difficulties in complete silence. So go for the sympathy vote!

Then having explained your condition to others, you may find that the biggest surprise of all will come. Your friends especially will start to tell you about the time when something awful happened to *them* and even when they lost some hair or someone else they know had a similar problem. Many will want to confess something or other to you. Everyone may now have a story of a situation or condition that is so much worse than your own. Some will be relieved to feel able to talk to you as they assume you will be sympathetic.

Hair loss is much more common than people admit. It just needs everyone to start talking about it to make it more acceptable and better understood. It seems that the only ones who can do anything about this are the ones who are experiencing the problem for themselves, the very people who also find publicity the most difficult. Occasionally a magazine article will appear about hair loss, alopecia or similar conditions, but the editors will usually prefer to latch onto a story filled with emotion, rather than offering any really practical advice. After all, drama and emotion sell copies. Similarly, the rare television or radio programme on this subject will tend to touch on the raw medical aspects or on the new experience of an unusually vocal sufferer, rather than looking at the much longer-term impact on life and lifestyle. I hope to redress that balance.

4

Oh, is it a wig?

Somewhere along the line, someone is going to mention... wigs. Yes, *wigs*! Surely, the ultimate terror for any woman who has started to lose her hair. And I am not going to deny that it was with utter and tearful dismay that I viewed the prospect of having to wear one, not by choice but through apparent necessity. The people who said the words casually to me 'You can always try wearing a wig' might just as well have been saying 'nice weather, isn't it?' for all the significance the prospect seemed to mean to them. But for me they were words never to be forgotten and indeed they still echo in my thoughts.

I used previously the words 'having to' wear a wig because plenty of people wear wigs voluntarily, for modelling, for doing anything in the public eye, for parties, for character performances on stage or on television. I often wonder how they would react if they found they had to wear a wig every day of their lives, all day, and in all circumstances. I also feel very angry inside when jokes are made about the subject, although there are so many different ailments in life that it would be impossible to avoid every subject that might upset some minority or other.

There are many words and phrases in life that are used without a second thought, but which can cause upset to certain groups. In the case of a hair loss sufferer, a casual comment such as 'keep your hair on', used when someone is getting irate, has a rather more poignant meaning to someone struggling with alopecia. My own problem has made me much more careful about what I say to others, just in case they have a difficulty about which I am not aware.

Now as a long-term wig wearer, I have also observed an interesting phenomenon. Even when a friend feels that a new wig style or colour looks great, many do not know what to say by way of a compliment. Having someone apparently look at your hair but say nothing at all can be an uncomfortable experience, because the natural reaction is to think that they are silent because there is something wrong. In a nice turning of the tables, they may actually need help to talk to a sufferer about it. Indeed, I once received a spontaneous and highly complimentary reaction about my 'hair' from a person who definitely did not know that I was wearing a wig. Then, having explained the situation to her, she admitted that if she had known the truth then she might not have said anything at all.

It also seems that the very word 'wig' has certain connotations. I should very much like to propose the adoption of a new term that makes it all sound more positive and fashionable, such as 'hair enhancer' or 'style topper' (my copyright, I said it first!). It may be a long process though, as the word 'wig' is firmly entrenched in the manufacturing, supply and fashion industries.

At the hospital

The term sometimes used by the commercial wig suppliers for someone like me is a 'necessity wearer', that is, someone who has no realistic and practical option but to wear one of their 'wigs' to cover up the results of serious hair loss. At the time when first I had to resort to these, I was still undergoing medical investigations, so acquiring one became a matter of obtaining an 'appliance'. This latter term made the whole thing seem so much worse. An appliance for goodness sake! Could there not be a better description? There was a degree of form filling to go through, followed by a visit to the hospital department dealing with every appliance from crutches to artificial arms. I had not had an accident, nor had I been born with or acquired what would normally be understood as a disability. I was not ill. I did not want to be there. When the person behind the desk asked about my application, with other patients in earshot in the waiting room, I was absolutely devastated.

When I was left for a moment in a large consultation room, feeling utterly vulnerable, I was mortified when someone else came in by mistake and saw me wigless. The staff did not seem to mind, but I did. More than they will ever know. Their unintentional 'insensitivity' had a very negative effect on the way I felt at that time and I am sure that as caring people they would have been most unhappy if they had realised this.

Then the next move was to return to the hospital for yet another appointment to see a lady who carried a small supply of wigs in a 'suitcase' from which I could select and place an order. It seemed almost rather furtive. What she had was a very small choice and the styles were not for me at all. For chemotherapy or other medical patients who may need urgent and immediate hair care assistance, especially whilst staying in a ward, this service is wonderful and invaluable. But I would suggest to the medical profession that for those outpatients facing an ongoing hair loss condition it might not be an entirely appropriate solution. More advice on suppliers outside the hospital would have been really helpful and might also have saved valuable healthcare time and paperwork.

Some years after the initial experience, still the only advantage I can see in going through this humiliation is to get a little off the cost of buying a wig, either via prescription or the exemption of a local purchase or sale tax - but I have more to say about tax in a moment. Others may have a far happier hospital experience, but mine was unfortunate and pretty much put me off seeking medical assistance for the condition forever. Fortunately, in my own domestic situation and taking into account the money saved long-term by not having to pay hairdressers' bills, I was able to pursue an alternative and private purchasing option. After all, like it or not, in the UK the National Health Service's financial assistance does not cover the whole cost of a reasonably good wig. Personally, I think this is appalling. Although I was treated as if I was in some sort of disability category, I had (and still have) no real financial help for this long-term and costly medical condition.

If you have only a minimal budget, be reassured that there are plenty of lovely styles around and you will always be able to find something to suit. Going up the range with wigs works exactly the same as it does in any high street shopping expedition. There's something good for everyone, whatever the circumstances. Paying a lower price does not necessarily mean that you do not look good, although the durability and overall quality of a purchased item may evidence itself in the longer term.

Shopping around

After a while, and having gained more confidence, I wanted to expand my choice of wigs. My husband and I were absolutely certain that there must be plenty of suppliers that we could consider. Some towns have high street wig shops where you can walk in, have a look around, see the goods, buy and walk away. A few of the large indoor shopping complexes or markets have stalls selling ladies' wigs. This sounds simple to most people, until it is realised that in order to try on a wig in such a place then the existing hair deficiency has to be 'exposed' in full. It is rather like looking at forbidden fruit. I knew what I wanted and there were shops that stocked the goods, but how could I get my hands on them?

I would urge you not to worry too much about this though. As I was soon to discover, a good wig shop will always be able to offer complete discretion in having a private room for trying on a selection of styles and colours, and will have an experienced and sensitive member of staff to assist. It might also help to know that a supplier may use the term 'postiche' (meaning false) and that 'piece' is sometimes used to refer to a ladies' wig, although this might also refer to an add-on or clip-on extension rather then a full head covering. Many shops also offer a service whereby a home visit can be arranged for complete privacy. Perhaps a partner or friend would be prepared to make an initial enquiry on your behalf, or to accompany you to a shop to provide some support?

The people who attend the hospitals to supply wigs are sometimes wearers themselves, or have known someone with hair loss. They may have their own specialist business or be part of one of the shops mentioned above. If you can find out where their main base is located, it is a really good idea to try to meet them there. That way you can get to see much more of the stock. Most would prefer to meet you too, so that they can have a better understanding of your needs and have an opportunity to give you the very best service. The atmosphere can be so much more relaxed and choosing a wig can actually become quite fun. It is absolutely amazing how different styles and colours can change one's personality. Always fancied being a different colour but never had the courage to see what it might look like? Want something more glamorous for the evenings?

Finance and Tax

Many of the UK suppliers are registered for charging Value Added Tax (VAT) and will be able to exempt this from purchases made in the UK if you are a genuine necessity wearer. In other countries there are various modes of financial assistance and varying regulations regarding purchase taxes. The possible deduction of any costs is perhaps one positive reason for going through those early stages of hospital visits, just in case there is a need to demonstrate a background that can prove necessity circumstances if required. In almost all instances, you may simply be asked to complete and sign a very short form when you buy your wig, the emphasis really being on providing the supplier with something for his or her own paperwork that shows a price has been discounted legitimately. However, it is important to realise too that if you are a necessity wearer then you are eligible not to pay the VAT element of a wig's price under any purchasing circumstances, so in my view you should consider avoiding any supplier who does not offer this up front or when asked.

How many to buy and what to expect

Expect to buy an average-quality fibre wig two or three times a year, more times if they have heavy wear and tear - and of course more if you simply want a range of styles. With care, a more expensive real hair wig may last up to two years. However, most women would naturally want to change their hairstyle before that. It is quite usual to collect a range of styles and types over time and ringing the changes between them does of course prolong the life of each individual wig. They will usually come in neat and discreet packaging or small boxes, sometimes wrapped in tissue paper and/or a protective net, and these can be placed neatly within a cupboard, wardrobe or dressing room. It is pretty much the same as storing shoe boxes. A mail order supplier will almost certainly use plain wrapping or labelling that will be highly unlikely to convey the nature of the contents to anyone else.

A growing number of suppliers have catalogues which they will mail to you so that you can browse at leisure, although, with the best will in the world, as printed documents these can never be comprehensive or entirely up to date. Always check back before ordering that your choice is still available and at the same price. Others do prefer customers to make more personal contact anyway, because the stocks and styles change rapidly and it is very difficult to make safe recommendations without seeing an individual's facial shape and skin tone and discussing style preferences. Several suppliers now also offer their wigs for purchase via the Internet, keeping the whole thing exceptionally private. Some of these also offer to arrange the VAT deduction, whilst others might try only to give a smaller (but reasonable discount) to necessity wearers or repeat buyers. It is always your choice entirely.

Internet shopping

If you are a computer Internet user, do a web search and have a browse at what is out there. You can ask questions by email or by telephone and goods will be sent in discreet packaging. A reputable outfit will have a website with all terms and conditions clearly displayed and will take credit card payments under secure conditions. Check the terms and conditions of your credit card as you may find that paying a supplier with a card for more expensive items gives you some comeback via the credit card company if things go wrong.

You may also wish to ask your supplier how any purchase will appear on your credit card statement, especially if someone else is likely to see that statement. Some suppliers use a word or series of initials that offer far greater discretion than others. Those that do will also be more likely to exercise most discretion in other aspects of their supply work.

Many mail or Internet order suppliers will take back unsoiled and unused returns if the chosen item is faulty or is really genuinely unsuitable, though it may only offer an exchange rather than a refund and will probably expect you to pay or contribute to postage or 'admin' costs. Some will only accept returns if the item has barely been touched, let alone tried on for fit. Others may require a small 're-stocking' fee of some kind. But that is really not so different to many other commercial transactions for other types of product. Check the terms and conditions carefully before you order.

Using the Internet can be a really excellent way to extend your access to styles, colours and suppliers, once you are certain of what you really want. However, remember that not all colours look the same on different computer monitors, set-ups and printers. It is extremely difficult for any supplier to convey correct colour hues onto every screen setting and any such on-screen swatches must be viewed with caution. When you cannot try on the wig before buying, it may be best to go for a generally interesting colour, rather then putting too much emphasis on a very precise tone. If you have some hair, you might be able to ask your supplier to match a suitable wig colour to a sample piece of your own hair. You can also ask to see (or sometimes buy) sample colour swatches, and again a good supplier will be more than happy to send colour samples. Then there'll be less chance of a mistake or disappointment.

If you're good with things digital, or know an understanding friend who is, it is possible to take a photograph of yourself and using appropriate software then superimpose different wig styles over it to see what you might look like in different styles and colours. A wig that looks great on a smiling and professional model may look very different on you. I have often been really surprised to find that a wig I did not like much on a model looks great on me, and vice versa.

It's nothing unusual

Sorting all this out is not always a great experience but it has to be done. However, it is useful to bear in mind that the suppliers you deal with in this respect are doing the job of providing wigs for ladies every day. Thousands and thousands of them. They do not see it as anything unusual, so neither need you. Ask for their help in choosing. The smaller businesses, often run by experienced and very caring ladies, usually love their role and genuinely want to help each individual. Get to know each other and ask for recommendations. They may also alert you to suitable new styles as they are introduced.

If you can start to see the buying of a wig as being just the same as researching and buying any other clothes, then you will feel much more comfortable with exploring the options, checking out the marketplace, assessing the competition and knowing your consumer rights. The wig business is just another commercial operation. There are a few out there who just want to make money from your misfortune, but happily they are very few and far between. And finally, keep a sharp look out for those who advertise 'sale' prices and 'discounts', when the original price might already have been the same or lower before the sale.

5

Which wig to choose?

Having accepted that there is nothing for it but to wear a wig, where should you start? It is not something that most women have been brought up to see as normal and a wig is certainly not on the average shopping list. There are so many new things to learn about. Then once a supplier (or suppliers) has been identified, the range of wig brands, styles and colours can then be just as extensive, daunting and confusing. Just as you think you have found the very thing, another set of styles and colours presents itself. Yet over time you can also see this as rather exciting, offering a wonderful choice.

There are a number of tips I can give based on my years of very real and very practical experience. Perhaps the first thing to bear in mind is that there is definitely going to be a wig out there that will really suit you and one on which you will come to rely. It can be a shaky experience when the first few that you try on make you look and feel like a frump or a monster. This is perfectly normal. Decide that this will probably happen but that you don't ever need to accept anything permanently that has this effect.

Do not always take on board what the salesperson says – you would not (or should not!) when buying anything else. Unless you feel entirely happy with the item then it's a complete waste of money as you will end up leaving it in the box in a cupboard. Wigs really can look and feel absolutely fantastic, sometimes even better than having your own original hair (yes, really), so be persistent and accept nothing that threatens to chip away further at your confidence.

Another point to remember is that a new wig will be just that – new. It will need to be worn in, in the same way that a new pair of shoes might seem at first to be a little tight or stiff. Some of my all time favourite wigs have been those about which I was very unsure at the beginning. When they are first taken from a box or lifted off a stand they can seem quite alien. They need to shake down, to settle down, to mould to your own head contours and to fall in harmony with the pattern of your usual brush strokes.

Sometimes a wig does not even become 'you' until it has been washed for the first time. I will usually wear a new wig around the house for a few days, returning to an older one to go out, until I am happy that the new one has become a part of me. So do not be too dismayed if your choice appears at first to be 'sitting' a little too high, be too 'volumised' or not quite the right shape. It is still possible to make it your chosen and best purchase. In fact given just a little time it will feel really strange not to be wearing it.

Suppliers

With many other 'medical' conditions, and the various items supplied to deal with them, manufacturers and distributors concentrate their efforts on the health care marketplace and understand quite well all the special sensitivities of their customers and patients. However, with the wig industry, it may seem to the customer that medical needs are sometimes more of an offshoot from a far bigger commercial and non-medical playground that is its first priority.

For example, if you search on the Internet you may come up with anything from serious discussion of hair loss, and recommended treatments and medications, to fantastical wigs as part of theatrical costumes, from caring alopecia help groups to magnificent hair creations as part of the sex toy industry. This can be upsetting for anyone coming to terms with the unwanted condition of hair loss and doing research for the first time. Seeing wigs sold as optional or rather 'fun' items often makes me feel resentful and it feels as if my own affliction is thus being 'trivialised', even though this is entirely unfair on perfectly legitimate businesses serving their own customer base. On the more positive side, one might also comment that if wigs are something that non-hair-loss-sufferers sometimes want to get hold of, then perhaps wearing one out of necessity cannot be all that bad after all.

Try not to be put off by all of this commercial marketplace stuff. If anyone has a style and colour of wig that you want, then buy it. Internet suppliers may never meet you face to face and it does not matter where the wig comes from if it helps you to deal with your life. However, you might want to look for the option to tick a box on a website screen to makes sure that your name is not added inadvertently to 'inappropriate' mailing lists. Of course this advice applies to any product shopping

Just as with any manufactured product, a number of suppliers will sell the same items under the same or even a different product name. Take time to make your comparisons. In my long experience of buying wigs, whilst most of them maintain similar prices to one another, others can vary considerably for the same product description. They may also vary delivery charges, guarantee periods or willingness to accept returns, so just go with the supplier that appeals to you the most. Only very occasionally will you find a really substantially cheaper offer for the exact same item, so making a purchasing mistake in this context is not going to be a big problem.

As mentioned earlier, there are many high street shops selling wigs and hairpieces and some will cater for the necessity wearer and the need for privacy, whilst some will not. You need to look around your own area. If you can, start with the recommendation of your medical consultant, general practitioner or nurse, and work out from there as you become more experienced and more confident. Remember though, if you want to have a tax deducted from the cost of your purchases, you may need to be ready to give the name of your 'medic' to your wig supplier if required.

Partial wigs

For those who have temporary or partial hair loss it might be possible to resolve the situation by using clip-on, pin-on, or interwoven hairpieces and extensions. These can be woven or plaited into head hair for an excellent and well-disguised effect. The colours can also be matched extremely well to own hair colour. Remember though that if you have dyed your own hair, as it grows out from the roots the colour of hairpiece needed may need to change accordingly.

For the more confident or fashion-conscious, having a range of hair extensions can be highly desirable and can be contrasted deliberately with own hair colouring. Extensions are often used enthusiastically by those without any own hair loss at all. They are chosen to dress hair for a social occasion using bright colours or plaited strands – or just for the everyday pleasure of it.

Later I will be looking at how part wigs and small pieces can be attached under a cap or hat, so usefully the wearer then appears to have a full head of hair underneath it.

Full wigs

The ranges and makes of full wigs are extensive and can be very confusing to the reticent and uninitiated. Some manufacturers and suppliers also have a penchant for quoting their styles and colours as a series of instantly forgettable numbers. Others use their own choice of names for styles supplied under other names by a competitor outlet. This gets even worse when blends of colours are used, with different numbers and names for shades of others. It is best not to get too 'bogged down' with these and just go for the colour that appeals to your eye, noting the reference number though in case later you want to re-order.

There are literally hundreds of styles out there, mostly mass-produced in the Far East on machines and most commonly using artificial fibres. It is a very highly sophisticated and well-established industry. The simple rule here is that you get exactly what you pay for. The cheapest wigs will be the poorest quality, perhaps in their construction, in their expected durability during wear (you do not want the fibres to fall out in the same way as you lost your hair!), or in degrees of excellence of styling. Unfortunately, each will cost more than an average single trip to the hairdressers, so do be prepared to have to pay out, but then you may need less wigs in a year than you would have needed haircuts so things do even out eventually. When starting out, it may be a good idea to buy a fairly modest wig, or more than one if you can afford it, so that you can get used to what you like best and how to manage it. Expect to get through several styles before you can fix on one that becomes a favourite.

Although many wigs are machine-made, in my experience they may not always be exactly the same as each other when they come off the production line. This could be because many different machines are being used at the same time or because the same pattern is made at different factories. Hand-made or hand-finished wigs will also be dependent on the skills of the individual worker. Also in my experience, this means that if you re-order a wig of a favourite style and colour, it may turn out to be a little better or worse than the one previously purchased. In one case I had to return a wig as being styled in way that was so far different from the previous one of the same reference number as to be unrecognisable as the same style, though fortunately this is rare these days. Just be prepared. Wigs vary - and you're paying. It might be a good idea to choose something different every time you re-buy. That is more fun anyway.

You have a good choice of wig construction. It is now possible to be quite selective, choosing a wig where some or all of the fibres are affixed to a lightweight scalp-coloured cap. This means that it appears so much more like real hair than the cheapest wigs, allowing styling in different ways or to be parted in a breeze to reveal 'skin' at the top rather than threatening to show some kind of fabric meshing. Often referred to as 'monofilament' or 'skin top' wigs, these are really the best to seek out if you can afford to pay a little more. Once you have had one you'll probably never want anything else. Furthermore, some wigs have a dual construction, been part machine manufactured and part hand knotted or hand finished.

The more expensive fibre wigs will give you a better quality of overall styling, in just the same way as a better hairdresser would give you a better haircut. The production techniques and varieties of product have leapt forward in the time that I have been wearing wigs and the main suppliers now keep up with all the latest hair colour trends and fashions. There is absolutely no need to look unattractive in a wig. In fact it can be very much the opposite case, so easy is it to switch to a brand new 'you' and to look and feel really great. In fact, prepare yourself for plenty of compliments.

Fibre wigs

The term 'fibre' wig is generally used for anything that is not made of real human hair. Be assured that these days fibre (synthetic) wigs can be so good that it is often difficult to tell unless very close up that they are not real hair. Furthermore, if you look and act 'normal', then as no one is expecting you to be wearing a wig they will not be looking closely for this. There are clever blends of colour and texture to suit all tastes, there are short and long styles, straight and curly, modest and exotic, everything to suit the young and the not so young.

If you do not see what you want then ask to see some catalogues and then ask to see some colour swatches for the chosen style. A good outlet will be prepared to get hold of a few items from which you can make a selection without obligation to buy any of them. If you are doing this in a shop, make sure you get chance to see yourself in a mirror wearing the wig from a distance and viewed from every possible angle. It is exactly like choosing a dress or a new pair of shoes. You will learn to look forward to and quite enjoy the experience as your confidence grows.

Make sure that you check the colours in natural light as well as under artificial lighting. These can be quite different, just as with any fabric or manufactured colouring. You have to like the colour in all conditions. Again, it's just like choosing any other item of clothing. You might also want to try a wig colour against the colour of your favourite earrings, often-worn clothes or usual spectacle frames. Remember too that some wigs will lose a little of their colour intensity with wear, washing and sometime with exposure to very strong sunlight.

Perhaps one of the most difficult things is trying on a likeable style but not feeling able to go home with it because it is in the wrong colour. You will be able to order other colours, but it is so hard to imagine what it will really look like on you until you have both the chosen style and colour together. Similarly, do not choose a colour on a stand but then dismiss it because the style is wrong. Your supplier will be able to help you achieve the correct combination. In many ways it can be even better than having your own hair. You can change your look instantly or dress in a moment for going out. Though the disadvantages of hair loss often seem overwhelming, this can be balanced out a little by recognising some of the real advantages.

It may sound blatantly obvious, but fibre wigs do not grow. What you see is what you get. The style you buy is usually the style you keep. The real temptation with an almost-right style is to get the scissors out and trim a bit here and there, especially around the fringe area. Don't! It never works well and there is absolutely no going back. The fibre wigs are styled to be exactly as you see them. Fibre wigs certainly can be trimmed, but get your professional supplier to do it for you. Not only will they do it properly, but also if it goes wrong you have some redress. If you do not like the fundamental style when you first put it on, allowing for settling in, then you will never be able to change it substantially. I have bought a particular wig and then felt dreadful in it, but had to wait weeks until I could budget for another one. This does more than anything to sap confidence and self-esteem. If you're not entirely sure, try another one. The rule is style first, colour second, trimming (by experts) only if absolutely essential.

Most fibre wigs are constructed using a kind of appropriately coloured webbing or mesh cap into which the separate fibres are stitched or knotted. It should be remembered that even with the best wig-making techniques, it is always only a manufactured product and not original scalp. There will be some imperfections, even with the very best example, though usually the foundation work is well concealed in the finished items. Sometimes on cheaper wigs there is too much fibre thickness making the wig look and feel bulky, or perhaps there will be some very visible cut ends spiking up at the crown. Have a look at the crown of the wig and all along any partings and make sure that at least this appears to be minimal. Do not be afraid to reject a wig and order up another of the same specification, because, as I said before, they can vary.

Real hair wigs

The ultimate dream for most wig wearers, other than getting one's own hair back of course, is surely to have a real hair wig. They are lighter and more comfortable and of course only real hair looks like real hair. Only real hair moves and falls like the original. Only real hair feels like the real thing, from the wearer's point of view and also perhaps from the view of the wearer's partner. The latter may be a very important consideration and should not be overlooked, and particularly if someone less than sympathetic is involved.

However, some people have an understandable aversion to the idea of having hair that once belonged to someone else. I had always dreamed of progressing to a real hair wig. After really liking a real hair wig when I eventually acquired one, to my great surprise I soon developed almost a revulsion to the idea after a very short time. Although it was human hair I could not make it feel anything like my own. It was almost as if I had someone else with me and also I didn't like to imagine what had happened to get it to me. I suppose this is something akin to the psychological difficulties that an organ transplant recipient might sometimes feel, although of course the circumstances are rather different because wig-wearing is non-intrusive and not due to a life-threatening situation in the general context.

Some people may be prevented from wearing a real hair wig, or a wig from a particular type of source, due to various religious, cultural or political concerns. Any supplier or carer should make themselves aware of this possibility and the importance to certain groups of adhering to their family or community beliefs or restrictions. Not to do so may cause great offence and upset.

In their defence, a real hair wig may be a combination from many different sources and will have gone through all sorts of preparations since origination. A necessity-wearer will also have a very genuine, quasi-medical requirement that can be said to put one in a different category to the usual high street or vanity consumer. Go ahead if it's real hair you want, can have, and can afford it, but always remember the same rules. You get the quality of hair, quality of manufacture and quality of styling that you pay for. Find out what the current typical price range is for a real hair wig (much more than most fibre ones) and go as far up the range as you possibly can.

In just a few cases where hair loss is predictable, perhaps due to planned medical treatment or known family tendencies, or where only a small part of the head is affected in the longer term due to scarring, then it might be possible to utilise one's own hair. Long hair in particular can be cut in advance of a predictable problem and can then be fashioned by a skilled wigmaker into a real hair wig, extension or piece using the sufferer's own source hair.

If you are often with small children, especially babies, then it might be better to look at the 'pros and cons' of a real hair wig over a fibre one, or a very high quality soft and fine fibre wig over a cheaper version. Anything that gets near to a very small child's face should be as soft as possible. Similarly, a short, close fitting style might be less of a temptation than a long one to a grasping child's hand. Incidentally, always be prepared for children to make spontaneous and sometimes 'hurtful' comments. They will not have acquired the art of tact!

Generally speaking, real hair wigs do require more daily management than fibre ones, especially after washing. More about this later.

Size and fit

Ladies' wigs usually come in two head sizes, petite and average. A good supplier will want to take your head measurements and some will create bespoke items (at a price). You can also find out from some suppliers, including those on the Internet, how they advise you to take your own head measurements using a fabric tape measure. It is best to check with your supplier to make sure what criteria they are using for a particular manufacturer's products. As a general rule, not many ladies will need petite. The average sizing suits most people, although some with total hair loss might just find the reduced size suitable and more secure if not too tight. As a necessity wearer I still find the average size is generally most comfortable.

In the overwhelming desire to achieve a feeling of maximum security, it is important that you do not purchase a wig that is going to be too tight or cannot be adjusted. A wig that is too tight will cause headaches, or worse, in the same way that you would never wear a hat that was too small or constricting. A tight wig, when removed, will also leave unsightly red lines on delicate scalp areas, like the result of wearing a pair of firmly-elasticated socks. A well-fitted wig should always feel comfortable and light, as well as secure, so that after a while the wearer can almost forget about it being there.

There may also be sales descriptions such as precise dimensions of 'bangs', 'crown' and 'nape'. This can be daunting. Check how your chosen supplier describes these and measures them, but usually 'bangs' means the length of the fringe strands down from the top where they are tied, the crown is the length from the top of the head to the base of the wig at the back and the nape is the length of the hair that falls from the bottom edge of the wig at the back and down the neckline.

The wigs can be adjusted once you have them, so if an average size wig is a little too loose, or works loose with wear, then it can be tightened. This is done by adjusting either the concealed 'sticky' fabric tapes integral to the base of the wig, or the discreet tapes and hooks, the type depending on the manufacturer and style. This works a bit like altering an adjustable skirt waistline. You can achieve a very secure and comfortable fit that is unlikely to move about unless tugged.

There are new developments coming along all the time. It is now possible for someone with total hair loss to have a quality wig affixed semi-permanently to the scalp (sometimes using a tightening vacuum effect), enabling normal washing, swimming and general activity whilst wearing a wig yet without fear of dislodgement. For many this gives the freedom and confidence that can enhance their lives dramatically, though it comes at a price.

Better still for the average wig wearer with a little or almost none of her own hair is a development, which personally I find an absolute wonder. On the inside of some wigs you will find machine-sewn pieces of a special transparent or suitably coloured polypropylene material, which adheres to warm skin. Anyone who wears a wig will know how warm things can get. With this stuff, the warmer the head, the more secure the fit. Combine wig wearing with menopausal hot flushes (and many ladies suffer this 'little' problem!), or with active sports or being in a hot atmosphere, then you have a remarkable solution to the fear of unscheduled wig movement that gives the only advantage I know to having 'hots'. The inclusion of this material really is a feature to look out for and I cannot recommend it highly enough. If your chosen wig does not have it in already, ask your supplier if it can be added. They should be able to have it hand sewn in for you for a modest additional charge. It is really worth it. Face the breezy days with confidence again. I'm not sure how well it would stand up to a grasping child, but it will certainly restore your confidence to go out on a windy summer day or be close to others in a crowded place.

Weights

It is surprising how much variation there can be between different wigs in terms of how much they weigh. I have often wanted to throw one off in frustration, especially on a hot day. Weight of wig can make such a difference regarding levels of comfort. Obviously, a longer wig is likely to weigh more than a shorter one, but different types of hair and fibre, as well as different types of construction, can also make quite an impact. Some makes of fibre strand are also finer than others, so two seemingly similar styles can have quite a difference in weight.

A certain amount will depend on whether you are choosing a partial or a full wig. Obviously a full wig will usually weigh more than an extension. However, contrary to some beliefs, it is not true to say that a lighter weight full wig will necessarily be less secure than a heavier, fuller one, or that a short one will be less likely to move about than a longer one. After all, a big, thick woolly hat can be pulled off just as quickly as a small, thin cotton one!

For security, the most important aspect is fit. For comfort, the important aspects are fit and weight. Check with your supplier about the weight of a wig before you buy it. This can also help you to make a decision between one or more styles. When you have found a favourite, make a note of its weight and keep this in mind as a comparison against anything else you may buy in the future.

Matching your skin

Although everyone knows that their own hair may lose its colour as they get older, others do not always appreciate that their skin will also change its tones over the years. For instance, a strong, dark hair colour on a younger woman with fair skin might look false and unattractive on her when she becomes much older. Nature (left to its own devices) might by now have selected a lighter, softer tone.

It may be that the longer-term wig wearer will wish to consider this when selecting a series of wig colours over time. This will depend very much on her personal approach to her situation, whether she is wishing to conceal her hair loss from others or fight back with a bold 'so what if I am' fashion statement. After all, presumably she would not see anything unusual in modifying her makeup, lipstick or own hair colour as she matures.

Having originally had quite dark and reddish hair, as time progressed I started to choose wigs that were a little more on the 'brown-blonde-grey' side of things. However, I got it wrong and had moved away from a colour a little too early, the lighter colours tending to age and drain my skin's natural appearance. I moved to something more akin to a warm blonde and then back to my original darker colour. But the good thing about wigs is that it is the easiest thing in the world to change them, whereas dying your own hair and making a colour error is a bit more difficult and untimely to rectify.

Think about the general colour image you wish to convey, the different lighting situations in which you may wear your wig, and whether you might want eventually to assemble a selection of colours for different occasions, moods and ages. You can have an enormous amount of fun with this.

Styles and lengths

Everyone has their own preference regarding style and length and many who have to wear a full wig wish only to replicate the chosen appearance of their original hair. This may also be because they want to conceal the fact that they are wearing a wig and want to look much the same as usual. Or perhaps a partner prefers the original style. Of course this makes selecting a wig style much easier as you know exactly what to choose. Most basic styles of women's hair are available in wigs and manufacturers are quite good at serving fashions.

However, it might just be time for a bit of a change, especially if you used to have very long hair. A long wig, especially a fibre one, might introduce unforeseen problems. Tying it back with bands or clips can damage the fibres quite quickly. Putting it up into a 'bun' or 'tail' can open up the possibility of exposing the meshing at the edge of the neck. So it is wise to think through how you would usually wear your 'hair' if you do prefer a longer length.

If you enjoy an outdoor or very active lifestyle it might be best to look for a shorter style. This may not be your first choice if it was your own hair, but in being easiest to manage it could prove to be less of a problem in the end. Wearing a wig is one thing, but introducing new concerns is to be avoided.

Layered, spiked or 'scruffy' styles can be the most effective because real hair is rarely super neat. Some fibre wigs are particularly good at responding to fluffing them up with your fingers, or changing the style as a result of a different direction of brushing. Original real hair rarely looks exactly the same from one day to another.

Consumer assertiveness

Unfortunately the early embarrassments and numerous practical aspects of having to wear a wig make it difficult to put into practice the usual sort of consumer assertiveness, even for those who know the ropes. Buying a wig still *feels* different to buying a dress or a piece of furniture. However, it is so important always to bear in mind that you are a customer in a straightforward commercial selling and buying chain. People are making money out of your apparent misfortune, so make them work hard for their returns.

It is a good idea always to try to have someone else with you whose opinion you respect and who is prepared to speak up if you are in any way feeling hesitant or reticent. Give yourself plenty of time to choose and do not ever allow yourself to be hurried or persuaded against your instincts. Getting the right wig is supremely important and can change entirely the way you feel about yourself, the way you interact with others and the way you approach every day of your life.

6

Fashions

If only wearing a wig could be truly fashionable! Perhaps someone in the fashion industry could pick up on this thought and make wig wearing ('style toppers') more generally desirable beyond the catwalk or party, creating their own fortune out of it if they so desire, whilst we necessity wearers could become a great deal happier with our lot. It would not even be all that new an idea, for like all fashions it would simply be a re-invention of something that went before. But what a wonderful opportunity for a young designer to step in and make their mark in an area of fashion that is just waiting to be developed further.

History

It seems that human hair, having it or not having it, has long been a problem area. Learning a little about the interesting history of replacement hair helps to put wig wearing in a wider context and gives it a more open perspective. Wigs can be seen as part of an extensive and centuries old cycle of fashion trends as well as a kind of modern medical aid.

In ancient times in hot climates, some men, in valuing head hygiene, would shave their heads and wear a sensibly cooling and washable everyday linen headdress. For special dress wear, a natural hair or palm fibre wig would be worn. Young ladies might also shave their heads. In England for instance, by the 1600s long hair was fashionable for men, and those less well bestowed with natural hair would supplement their own with hair wigs. Trying to conceal the artificial pieces was abandoned completely by the mid-1660s and wigs became great outward fashion statements and status symbols. People actually wanted to wear wigs, something today's long-term wig wearer may find quite incredible.

Thus in the seventeenth century, wigs came to be highly prized by the most well-dressed citizen. But interestingly it was the men who continued to take the lead rather than the ladies, even wearing modified versions in the course of military duty. The diarist Samuel Pepys was hugely disappointed when his first wig wearing failed (he thought) to attract enough admiring attention. The wigs might be dyed and perfumed, to complement the glamour of a gentleman's finger rings, feathered hats and gauntlet gloves. Dress for the head was given more attention than other items of clothing, so much so that by the turn of the eighteenth century the affluent male would have his head shaved deliberately to accommodate a mountain of long and artificial curls costing the equivalent of many hundreds of pounds.

In hot weather, to help with the discomfort of the wigs, they might be tied back with ribbons, a style which became a more regular one by 1700, with embroidered caps worn privately at home. The less prestigious males would also wear wigs when possible, though they would be less flamboyant and look more like real hair. The very lowest classes would wear a short, small and plain item, a practice sometimes also adopted by the daring fashionable lady. Thus the twenty-first century lady need not feel that wig wearing is anything so very unusual.

It was a love of wigs that influenced the design of hats and gradually made them less important, so that whereas a man might once have kept his hat on his head when indoors he would now remove it on entering and carry it around under his arm. This is echoed in the twentieth century male good manner of removing a hat on entering a building, though appears to be dying out in the baseball-cap beginning of the second millennium!

We would surely see the once essential long, curly wigs for men as rather ridiculous nowadays, which just goes to show how fickle the whole fashion business can be over time. Fortunately, we now have an increasing acceptability of fashion wigs for woman, with an increase in shops that specialise. They are also popular amongst those with many other gender considerations who wish to amend their appearance. All we need now is one bright young designer to re-introduce them again as a real must-have fashion accessory for all. Many women with full heads of their own natural hair would surely cheer to be able to sport a gorgeous ready made style every day and every time of day, and many men would love to be able to have their hair so easily 'restored', both groups without fear of adverse 'wiggy' comments.

Changing perceptions

Many of the wigs around in daily use now are artificial and it is often considered either an expensive luxury to be able to wear a real human hair version or simply undesirable to wear another person's hair. Conversely, in the eighteenth century many wigs were made of real hair, though it wasn't always human. When neither human nor the cheaper horse or goat hair was available, or when something more sporting was required, then various duck feathers might be used, but naturally these were difficult to keep in good order and sometimes caught fire when the unfortunate wearer came too close to a naked flame. Other manufactured fibres might from time to time be used to make wigs, but not surprisingly the 'durable' copper wire or iron wigs that were introduced from Paris had a very short popularity!

Women did not miss out on all this activity. They would delight in adding extensions to their own hair, especially to the front to give extra height. This idea is believed to have been introduced accidentally when a lady out horse riding with Louis XIV tied up her windswept hair temporarily with a garter and was thus much admired, so did it again. All wanted to follow her example, even later using added lace and concealed supportive pads in this fashion craze. When the thick pads were believed to cause headaches, the real and the artificial hair were supported on lighter frames. Later the extensions moved to the back of the head, fixed with fearsome pins, and might be powdered along with the wearer's own hair. Some of the headdresses were adorned with objects such as a model ship or a miniature flower garden. Indeed, so large and complicated did some of the structures become that they were left unaltered for months, leading to infection and even living infestations.

One factor that helped to bring popular wig-wearing to a quick end in the eighteenth century was not any hygiene consideration, nor any dislike of the fashion, nor even any discomfort in wig-wearing, but rather the introduction in 1795 of a financial tax on hair powder. The powder had come into fashion in the 1690s. It was sometimes made of coloured as well as white starch and was used to keep the wigs dry, bug-free and sweet, whilst also offering opportunities for adding extra colour hues. The other major deterrent to wig wearing was the French Revolution when it ceased to be desirable to appear through exotic wig fashion to support or be part of the aristocracy. Wigs disappeared and hats started to return. It must have been a pleasant break for many who had long struggled with the heavy creations, but the necessity wig wearers of the day must have experienced much private distress.

Is having hair peculiar?!

Clearly then there has always been a desire in some cultures to adorn the head in one way or another, either with hair of a particular style, with a hat or with a wig. This might be done to protect the head from hot sun or other adverse weather conditions, to display colour or to symbolise wealth, to follow a short-lived fashion or to show respect.

If we regard only a shaven head as the true basic canvas, then even allowing real hair to grow might be seen as making an addition. After all, many women and even many men still go to great lengths to remove hair from other parts of the body, so why allow it to grow only on one particular area? Looked at in this way, displaying one's own head hair might be a rather peculiar thing! Indeed in some religions or cultures it is definitely not desirable to cut hair, whilst in others it may not be acceptable to let it be seen or to perceive it as a visible adornment.

If the question is asked as to why the head should be regarded as unusual, then it might also be advocated that wearing a wig is only one of a number of ways to dress the head, in the same way as we might alternate between dresses and trousers. Wig wearing in cultures where the display of hair is important should really not be seen as anything so very unusual. After all, few people with or shall we say 'wearing' their real head hair will feel that their hair is anything of great merit. Managing hair seems to be many a woman's daily problem. Just listen to everyone's complaints!

There are still some difficult areas today in the most open of societies where perceptions of vanity and necessity seem to overlap. Perhaps it is up to the wig wearers themselves to project a more positive image of the condition or preference? Instead of feeling disadvantaged or peculiar, we might see those struggling to manage their own hair as a rather peculiar and time-wasting activity!

7

Tricks and tips

S o now you have a wig. Lucky you. Yes, really, lucky you. Those eighteenth century wig-wearing men would have given anything to have access to the wonderful selection of styles, textures and fibres that are available to ladies today. You can look fabulous in a matter of seconds. Yet that first time out with it on can still be a tremendous ordeal. In today's society one feels as if the world is staring and making comment. They are not. Really they are not, but you will never be convinced easily. It seems as if there must be a large arrow pointing down at you to draw everyone's attention. You may feel as if the loss of your hair is the worst thing that could ever happen, when of course it is not. You may feel as if the next puff of wind will blow it off, which is unlikely but theoretically possible.

Before huge alarm bells start clanging, let me qualify that last comment. Anything worn that is not part of the human body can be detached in extremes of weather, be it a hat or a pair of sunglasses. To say otherwise would not be entirely honest. Yet the way wigs are made today, to fit and affix to the head so snugly, there is only the very smallest likelihood of any disaster. A minor movement might be the worst effect. The fear of discovery is by far the most difficult thing to tackle.

Windy days

On a windy day, with your own hair, you would either choose to let it blow freely or to protect it with a hat or a hood to safeguard your hairstyle. A wig can be treated in exactly the same way. In autumn or winter, wear a sweater, coat or jacket with a fashionable and acceptably styled hood. That way you can feel completely confident that should you find yourself in a windy situation you can take quick and evasive action. Knowing that this security route exists makes going out and about in adverse weather conditions so much easier. It is like driving along a motorway, but knowing that the side 'hard shoulder' lane exists to pull onto in an emergency.

Unfortunately, windy or breezy days in spring or summer are much more of a concern. To put a hood over one's head during a perfectly warm and sunny day, unlike everyone else around you, is of course likely to draw unwanted attention. This is an area with which I have long been worrying and wrestling. In my early days of wig wearing I was ignorant of how to address the problem and nobody gave me any useful advice. I have even resorted to wearing a headscarf for security on a windy beach overseas, which was fairly effective but made me feel atrociously old-fashioned as well as enormously self-conscious. It does work though and is better than any 'accidents', so I always have a snazzy chiffon scarf with me in a pocket for such trips. Worn with confidence, with a pair of fashionable sunglasses and designer shorts, a draped chiffon on an exotic beach can make you a bit of an incognito film star and will turn heads but for the 'right' reasons. But unfortunately this trick doesn't work at home in a busy shopping centre, nor is a suitable solution for some age groups.

Nowadays the manufacturers can offer a good range of hats with wig fringes, hats and trendy caps with long and short hair attached below, coloured shower-style turbans and suitably-shaped headscarves. There is a particularly good range of fashionable hats-with-hair for young children.

Think about various weather conditions when you are first choosing you wig style, especially with fibre versions. A fibre wig with a long fringe, however good it is, may have strands that can sometimes blow into the eyes. Unlike real hair, these can feel 'sharp' and as well as being supremely uncomfortable the repeated abrasion may damage the eyes. For this reason I have often resorted to having the troublesome fringe area of a fibre wig trimmed, which has to be done with extreme care so as not to ruin irrecoverably the manufactured style.

Security is the absolute key. If you feel the thing won't move, then you will feel so much better - and so will those around you who know about it. Try to buy a wig with the security inserts that adhere to warm skin. You can also use double sided sticky tape, one piece on the wig and a matching one on your skin, although personally I have never found this to be very satisfactory. If you have any hair at all, it might be possible to add extra security with slides and hairpins as I did in the earliest days of my problem, but unfortunately this is not an option that I can now enjoy.

Can I still go swimming?

Yes. Definitely.

One of my favourite pastimes is swimming and for many years before my hair loss my husband and I enjoyed a weekly swim. Then the hair loss presented a really major problem. How could I possibly continue to go to a pool where my wig would get wet? I was afraid that the whole wig might come off or might even float off if I got under the water? How would a wig react to the chemicals in the pool water? If it got wet would the foundation mesh start to show through? How could I go through the obligatory shower? I certainly could not appear without hair at all, or at least would not, although there are some who are prepared to do this.

Swimming is a real challenge. I tried out a series of swimming caps with very little success. Most caps were too tight to pull over a wig and in any case in doing so they made it move about. The rubberised materials were also a threat to the surface texture of the wig, causing damaging abrasion. If I wore only a basic swim cap, it was obvious that there was no natural bulk of hair beneath and these also pulled uncomfortably at my skin leaving red and sore marks afterwards. I did swim a few times in a classier cap with a fabric turban-style outer, but felt hugely self-conscious as of course no one else seems to bother with any kind of cap these days.

There are several solutions to this, one of which is *not* to stop swimming. Firstly, if you're lucky you can have your own pool, but most of us cannot! You could find a privately run pool in your area where numbers are small and there is less likelihood of being crashed into by boisterous junior swimmers. Alternatively, try to go to the municipal pool at the quietest times. Your wig will only be dislodged easily if you go right under the water and it is perfectly possible to have a great swim without submerging.

When you have been wearing wigs for a while, you will always have one that is getting worn out and is being replaced by a new one. Keep this and use it for swimming, changing into it in a cubicle before going to the pool and changing out of it whilst redressing. You can rinse and dry the swim wig at home and your everyday one has not been anywhere near the pool water (which may contain chemicals that could have an adverse effect on the texture of a wig). This works particularly well if you keep to one style as no one will know the difference. If you feel your after-swim 'hair' should have an authentic wet-at-the-ends look, then lightly dampen the ends or a wisp of the fringe with clean, cool water. If anyone else is about in the dressing area, this is easy to do with a quick pretend face wash at the hand basin in the changing rooms.

If you go swimming this in itself is a very good reason for choosing a fibre wig over a real hair one. A real hair wig will need to be dried and restyled if it gets wet, whereas a fibre one can be shaken and will dry naturally and usually very quickly. Managing a wet real hair wig in a changing room situation is just not workable without others being very well aware of the situation. Unless that is, you have been able to afford a bespoke and fully affixed product that can be wet and then dried on your head as if your own. However, being realistic, most of us will not be able to wear more than the 'ordinary' mid-range products.

If you are happy to wear a swim cap, another useful trick is to take an old wig and cut off the fringe and lower back pieces, then re-stitch these to the inside of a turban cap so they appear to be hair that is just not tucked in. This makes the cap itself easier to wear and can be very convincing. You might even be able to affix an entire wig inside a cap, especially a short one. Incidentally, this can also be done to any kind of outdoor hat, for instance to a sunhat for really hot weather or to a woolly hat in the winter. However, it should be said again that fabric hats could sometimes cause friction that can be damaging to fibre wigs, so I find it best to stick to the use of hoods in winter.

Choosing clothes

Trying on clothes in stores can be a nightmare, unless there are private cubicles, especially of course if they involve putting on and taking off items over the head. One major fear of wig wearers is that the item will move or become dislodged completely.

Fortunately the better retail stores usually have private cubicles now for trying on clothes. Be ready though for the over attentive assistant who might seem to be about to peep in and ask if you need any assistance. This is a good example of where it is best to have a thoughtful friend or partner with you when shopping. The assistant will usually be more than happy to leave them to do the reaching in and the fetching and exchanging of sizes.

Wearing a wig has certainly affected the clothes that I buy. I do prefer to choose items that do not have to go over the head, or ones that have unbuttoning or unzipping necklines, especially knitwear or tee-shirts. You never know when you might wish to remove a warm outer layer or put one back on, especially when going in and out of heated buildings in winter. Fashions that favour fleece jackets and loose items are very helpful. I also tend to avoid necklines that are fitted close in around the neck, as dressing and undressing will definitely dislodge the wig. Once these difficulties are recognised, it all becomes quite easy and instinctive. You will find yourself drawn naturally to the clothes that will make life as easy as possible.

Wigs that touch collars, or fall even longer onto clothing, can be damaged by friction. The result is that they go a bit frizzy and harsh at the ends, rather like bad split ends or dryness in original head hair. It does not look good and can make the wig much more uncomfortable to wear. This is not entirely avoidable. It can happen simply by leaning back regularly in a chair over a period of a few months. But the effects can be minimised by certain clothing fabric choices. Avoid too many synthetics and rough materials. Silk is always the least damaging. A short wig style can accommodate a raised collar much better than a longer one. The fibres on many a synthetic wig do not usually fall back into place once disturbed by a sticky-out collar, so think about the best combination for your fashion preferences and needs.

Having to wear a wig can also have advantages. One of these is having a great hairstyle ready to wear to go off to work, saving time and fuss in the morning, or for changing into in just a moment for going out in the evening. This is why building up a small collection of styles is useful. Also, where any lady with her own hair has to pull certain clothes over her head and thus leave her styled hair in disarray, in private you can pull off the wig, change your clothes and then put the beautifully arranged wig back on afterwards. Simple!

Can I wash my 'hair'?

Yes, you can.

You will be advised to wash your wig gently in tepid water, and not too frequently, using a specialist wig shampoo from a wig supplier. It was mentioned to me later that with care I could also use an 'ordinary' shampoo or liquid soap on a fibre wig, if the solution was a *very* mild and gentle one, followed by a little bit of a standard fabric conditioner, and rightly or wrongly I have found this to be very suitable. It also helps to add a pleasant perfume. In hot or dusty weather I have washed a fibre wig once or twice a week, whilst in some circumstances it might be enough to wash it once a fortnight (if away on holiday for instance).

A fibre wig usually comes pre-styled and will stay in that style wash after wash. This is the main advantage (other than, usually, the price) that these have over a real hair wig. All you need to do after final rinsing is to pat it dry in a towel, give it a gentle shake, and drape it over something narrow to dry naturally. You can buy a stand from your wig supplier and these are usually like polystyrene heads of the type that one might see in a fashion shop, or a plastic collapsible frame that can be carried in a suitcase for use in hotel rooms when travelling, but stretching a wet wig over a stand may stretch its fibres. You can always improvise something. The initial drip-drying can be done with the wig hung carefully over a bath tap. I have even used an upright kitchen towel holder. But a proper wig stand will help to restore the wig to the correct shape - when dry - and make it last longer. Its like any other item of clothing - the better the care, the longer its life.

Never brush a wet fibre wig as this damages it. It may pull the fibres from the 'roots' and cause 'hairs' to drop out and it may also damage the surface of the fibres. Brushing gently when dry is fine and in fact aids the restoration of the style.

Never use a hairdryer as it can 'melt' the fibres. You will not need to dry it with anything. Fibre wigs dry very quickly on their own. Incidentally, direct heat of any kind is always something to be wary about and I always keep a spare wig handy to wear when I am cooking using a fan oven. Avoid standing under heat sources, especially outdoor patio heaters. Needless to say, take care if you smoke and keep your wig away from sources of fire. In the event of a real emergency you can at least have the advantage of being able to throw off your 'hair' to avoid exacerbated skin burns.

Once the wig is dry (usually leaving it overnight in an averagely warm room will more or less do it), just give it another shake and a good brush. It will look great again, usually returning straight back to original style without any need to do any more work on it. It will feel cool, clean and good.

A real hair wig can be rather more problematic. It will usually come styled by a professional and thus will look absolutely fantastic at first. But although the hair is cut to a suitable shape and form, it *is* styled. When washed, the style falls, some doing so more than others. Remember how you would probably have needed to re-style your own hair with tongs, hot brushes or rollers after washing so this is quite a natural process. It should also be kept in mind too that the quality of hair may be even more variable than that found with manufactured fibres, all depending on the source hair, a straight real hair style perhaps becoming disappointingly frizzier or curlier when washed at home. The price you have paid may indicate what to expect, but there are no hard and fast rules. It simply is not possible for your supplier to tell you accurately what will happen to a particular wig until the first washing.

For this reason some suppliers may either try to deter you from buying a real hair wig or will recommend that you always return it for professional cleaning and restyling. In my view the latter is just too inconvenient. I feel that if you are capable and prepared to learn to wash and restyle your own wig then it is worth having a real hair version because they have the undoubted potential to look and feel the very best. Otherwise, the difficulties and inconvenience must be considered carefully according to individual needs, abilities and preferences. If you cannot re-style a real hair wig properly for yourself, then you'll feel much, much worse about everything than if you were wearing a permanently-styled fibre one. In that case, go for a top quality fibre product. After trying all options, the latter is now my preferred choice.

When formerly you styled your own hair, perhaps blow drying using a brush, the hair did of course remain in position attached to your head. Styling a real hair wig can be a little trickier as it needs to be held in place firmly so that the right kind of brush movement can be effected. Pull at it and the entire wig may follow. It can be maddening! I have found that with great care it *is* possible to blow-dry a real hair wig very well. Also, there are wig stands on the market now that have a special construction and heavy base, affording better opportunities for home styling to be successful.

Although the manufacturers might advise to the contrary, in my experience you can dry a well-fitting real hair wig from wet by placing it straight back on your head and working with it in the usual way, taking great care to hold any hairdryer at a good distance to dry it quite well before using a brush, and to brush *exceedingly* gently. Get a partner or friend to hold the dryer at a distance for you if you can, so that you can concentrate on the styling, using the brush with one hand and placing your other hand on your head to give some security. This is a bit of a performance at first, and if it all goes wrong it can be upsetting, but you can try again and you don't need to keep washing a real hair wig as often as naturally growing head hair. Once a week will do for normal wearing. It is just great to get that freshly shampooed smell back. Good for your partner too.

It may be worth bearing in mind that your supplier wants to keep selling wigs to you and if you buy a really good real hair version then you will return less frequently (though of course each less frequent purchase will be of greater value). If you can afford a real hair wig it can be worth pursuing. Be prepared for there to be quite a learning curve, but pursue it if you feel confident enough. My advice is for the averagely-skilled and averagely-financed wearer to start with manufactured fibre and progress to better quality versions, trying a real hair wig only as an 'extra' rather than go for this from the outset. Any difficulty with managing your wig in the early days will only make the whole problem of hair loss seem much, much worse.

Night time

Do I sleep in my wig?

That is entirely up to you and, where appropriate, up to your partner. It is certainly more comfortable to go without a wig in bed if you both feel accepting of this (and you can both get used to it as something quite normal), and if you're both asleep anyway then it should not matter! You can pop something on quickly in the morning if this aspect is difficult. Some wearers get so used to their wigs that they feel too vulnerable or even a bit chilly without one.

It is a good idea to keep an old wig of a suitable style if you wish to wear one at night, but do keep it clean and fresh smelling. That way you will not need to worry about wear and tear to your daytime wig from sweating or from pillow abrasion. If you do wear one at night then you will always want to have a fresh one ready for the morning. I have worn a spare wig when a patient in hospital and did not find any problems with this, although felt that I needed to advise regularly changing staff about it just in case. I also sometimes feel more 'safe' to have a night time wig to wear when away in hotels. Another option is to wear a well chosen and attractively designed turban or lightweight cap.

At home, always place your wig on a wig stand at night if you possibly can. This helps it to keep a good shape and also enables you to check visually that the styling at the back of the wig is in good order. If you want to conceal it or keep it dust-free, you can make an attractive cotton cover for the stand and wig, or perhaps loosely cover them with a bedroom-co-ordinating pillow slip if you are not too handy with the needle and thread. Use something that lets it all 'breath' but keeps it discreetly from view. This is not just an aesthetic thing. No one really wants to wake in the morning to see (in their half-waking) 'someone' apparently standing by the bed!

Heatwaves

I dread them. We have already talked about dealing with windy weather, but the most uncomfortable conditions for wig-wearers can be during a heatwave. Would anyone with their own hair ever contemplate wearing any kind of fabric or thickly made hat all day long when the temperatures soar? There is no doubt that wig-wearing is not desirous in these conditions, something also to be borne in mind when contemplating holidays to hot climates and beaches. So many times have I wanted to throw the thing off in a desperate desire to be free and cool, but of course etiquette and self-esteem prohibit this.

However, I have come across three possible solutions that have been really helpful. Firstly, in hot weather keep a spare wig in a separate container in your refrigerator, making sure of course that there is no chance of it becoming moist or picking up strong food smells. When you get hot in one wig, swap it over for a dose of cooling comfort.

Secondly, in private, take off the wig for a moment and wipe your head with lukewarm water. The slight warmth does not affect your overall temperature adversely, but the evaporative reaction of warm water on your hot head gives an instant cooling effect. On replacing your wig you may feel much refreshed for a while.

Thirdly, now available in many pharmacies and supermarkets are cooling adhesive gel pads designed specifically for applying in cases of mild fever. These work wonders if placed directly onto the skin under the wig. They are not likely to show through on lighter-coloured wigs or under monofilaments, although care may need to be taken if worn below a dark coloured wig or on darker skins. These will give an icy cooling effect for a few hours and I have found them remarkably good for keeping one's cool if going out in hot weather or for sleeping on a hot night. You can also get larger pillow-sized water and foam-filled pads as well. However, they may be unsuitable for certain medical conditions or for people liable to catch a chill, so everyone must make their own judgment on individual suitability.

In the privacy of your own home or in understanding company, and in really oppressive weather, there is always the alternative of a cotton cap.

Hot days are often sunny days. It is advisable to keep out of too much direct sun as eventually the heat and light combination may damage a wig. However, I have found though that usually the wig wears out naturally before any other factors cause damage. There is just the possibility that some wig colours can be affected adversely by continued strong sunlight, so sun worshippers should be mindful of this.

The choice of a monofilament or lightweight topped wig over any other kind is advisable if you are not someone who enjoys warmer weather. Any lighter construction of an item enables heat to evaporate more easily from the top of your head, as it would with your own hair.

Grooming on the go

In most circumstances wig hair is never entirely immoveable and may become disarrayed in wind or during any normal activity in the same way as real hair. Remember too that when a strand of a fibre wig blows up in wind it does not usually fall back down without help. Periodically run your hand gently over your head to make sure everything remains in reasonable styling. This is exactly what you would do if you had your own hair so it is not a big deal. There is no need to make it perfect, for what real hair is immaculate all the time? After all, a really perfect style is more likely to look like a wig than a ruffled one. Some wearers, especially the younger ones, will want to throw caution away and go for a super-fashionable fun wig, maybe in a 'shocking' colour, or perhaps with some trendy spikes or colour streaks, but few of us are prepared to go quite as far as that.

It is best to continue to carry a wig hairbrush with you when you go out (suitable for fibres), just as you did with your own hair. When you get chance you can give the wig a tidy here and there. Do be a little extra attentive in public though, as a loosely fitting wig might just move when pulled with a brush. A discreet placing of the other hand, just to hold the wig lightly in place whilst brushing, is perfectly easy to do and comes automatically with a little practice. You can also take the wig off in a cubicle, give it a refreshingly good shake and a little brushing before replacing it and re-emerging, and no-one needs be any the wiser. It can become easier to look good all of the time than it was to do so with your original hair. Some real hair wigs can also be restyled on the go if you wish, just like your own hair, using a handbag-carryable spray and a portable 'hot brush'. These accessories are useful on holiday when you do not want to wash your wig completely but it could do with just a bit of a lift.

Fibre wigs can sometimes smell a little less than fresh after continual daily wearing. In between washes, I find that a very, very light spray with a gentle wig or fabric freshener can help to give you that clean hair perfume. But go easy, both for reasons of not damaging the wig with an inadvisable chemical or 'sticky' reaction and so as not to attract the summer insects! But anything like that brushes out or washes out very easily.

Perhaps a 'safer' trick is to use a little of your favourite perfume on your scalp before putting on your wig. Again though, don't overdo it, as the warmth of your head under the wig may make the perfume too strong and can repel admirers rather than attract them. Also be careful of 'cheap' lotions and potions that may contain chemicals that could damage wig fibres. Warning: *never* put anything on your scalp that could cause burning, a real danger if enclosed or pressed down onto warm skin by the outer wig.

When I go on holiday, I always take a spare wig with me in addition to whatever I decide to use at night when sleeping. This means that if anything happens to one of them – and I bring to mind here the time a seagull's 'gift' just missed my hair and landed on my jacket shoulder! – you have something else to reach for quickly when you get back to the hotel without having to attempt a tricky washing and drying session. It is also great to be able to have a fresh wig that has not been worn all day so that you can change as part of dressing for dinner.

Eyes and makeup

There are probably more women around who have lost their eyebrows than there are those who have lost their head hair. This is because constant eyebrow plucking, or other forms of removal, can sometimes weaken the hair roots and eventually the brows may fail to grow back.

Where there are hairs remaining but they are fine or intermittent, it is quite easy to compensate by using normal eyebrow makeup along the existing eyebrow line. The difficult blank areas can be blended in with the real hair brows by using an eye shadow or cream applied with a soft brush and using gentle angled strokes. This is probably better than trying to draw in actual lines, which really only works well when done by an experienced makeup artist.

When all my own eyebrows had disappeared, I found that trying to redraw them back in was immensely difficult. Of course there was no longer a guideline to follow and the end results were never good. They also had a tendency to smudge or finish up looking unequal. The difficulty was compounded by my needing to wear spectacles for any kind of close work, which of course was impossible to do when applying makeup to the eye areas.

Then I discovered that I could have the eyebrows reinstated, or rather substitute eyebrows, using a form of semi-permanent eye makeup applied at a professional beauty salon. This was in effect a kind of tattooing, but simply with a series of exceptionally fine lines applied expertly and in a suitable colour. The proposed brow lines were drawn in with a special pencil first, to make sure that they would end up in the correct position. In my case, without any hair, they were also able to be slightly lifted from the original position on the 'maturing' face, thus adding a more youthful effect. So what a bonus!

I needed to attend for several sessions, not always very comfortable, and the brows were very sore for a few days afterwards so I had to choose a time when I could keep out of the social limelight. However, the effect is fantastic. I have been able to enjoy two perfectly groomed lines of eyebrows for several years now, without adding makeup. The treatment can be repeated when the new eyebrows eventually start to fade, although as I get older I prefer just a hint of a brow rather than anything that looks too heavy and 'new', and a little eyebrow pencil can always be applied to tone things up. I would strongly recommend the semi-permanent treatment to anyone without their own eyebrows, but of course only if you use a qualified and reputable practitioner.

After semi-permanent eyebrow treatment, it is vital to carry around a very high factor sunscreen cream, because bright sunlight will escalate fading of the new brows. You can buy a very small tube to carry in your handbag or car and make it a routine to rub a little on before walking about in the sun.

For those with a less severe hair loss problem, or those who prefer not to have such a dramatic treatment, there are now false eyebrows that can be purchased and affixed to the skin. You might wish to talk to a beautician about this, or to your wig supplier. Similarly, it has long been possible to buy false eyelashes, even through many high street chemists and at makeup counters, though personally I have not wished to use these despite losing most of my lashes.

The loss of eyelashes has been quite a difficulty for me, since with their departure also goes a level of natural protection for the eyes. Dust and infections can enter the body this way, which makes wearing spectacles preferable to wearing contact lenses as they offer a bit of a safety barrier. During the time when my lashes were falling out, not only did loose lashes trouble me regularly in my eye, but the red, itchy irritation along the eyelids was intensely uncomfortable. I discovered that this could be relieved by hand-splashing the eyes with a very mild solution of a tear-less baby shampoo mixed with plenty of water, in the same manner as washing the rest of the face. A medical adviser suggested that I could dab along the lids directly with this solution using a cotton bud, but I felt that there was a danger of any loose cotton fibres causing further irritation in the eyes themselves. Certainly though, establishing a careful cleansing regime is essential to avoid infection at the time when lashes are falling.

The loss of eyebrows and lashes will inevitably require a rethink of your eye makeup and it might be helpful to seek the advice of a qualified beautician to help you decide on a new way of working. Different parts of the eye are can be enhanced and emphasised and other parts made less noticeable. If you wish you can also discover new ranges of false eyelashes and even false brows. It's also a good excuse generally for some new makeup!

8

Getting on with it

C oming to terms with wearing a wig, especially if there seems to be no end to the timescale, is not easy. No one will pretend that it is. Even when it tries to be accommodating and understanding, modern society can be very tough on anyone who does not fit the perfect physical mould. It isn't going to be easy to change attitudes overnight.

The irony is that the very circumstances which would bring real and immediate sympathy (seeing you with no hair) are exactly the things that you will now do everything possible to avoid. You are highly unlikely to be seen or want to be seen without your hair or without your wig, other than by your closest partner or friend. Unlike a bandaged leg or a bruised face that can become displayable for effect, you must understand that those around you will try to be sympathetic but will find it really hard to understand what the problem is and what it really feels like. They have probably never seen on anyone this new phenomenon that you are talking about (and if you have anything to do with it they probably never will) so it is only realistic not to expect too much caring response back from them.

If you wish, one way to remind people constantly of your ongoing difficulty is to change your wig style and colour regularly, drawing some attention to the area of focus. Yet in these days of anything-goes-fashion, it is unlikely that many people will be much bothered by this. It is much better to accept your situation quietly, sort yourself out and then let yourself fall back into a perfectly normal life.

Friends may compliment you on your new style or even say how they almost envy you not having to struggle with wayward hair every day. Then they would rather not give it another thought and will hope to change the subject. Their envy may sometimes be genuine, but sufferers all know that nothing can compensate for losing a part of your feminine self. It is a fact of life that some women will lose their hair, and now it seems that you, or someone near you, is one of them. So you can either be down about it, or you can curse or say 'hey, it's tough, but it could have been something much worse'. Everyone is permitted a down sort of day and feeling upset and depressed about hair loss is perfectly natural. You should not regard any low feelings as unusual, in fact this is entirely to be expected. It does get better, a little bit more each day.

Changing one's appearance due to wearing a wig should be regarded as part of having a complete 'makeover'. When television programmes take on board an individual, analyse their deficiencies and then re-launch them to a fascinated audience, more often than not the main physical change is a new hair style or colour. Sometimes this would have been pretty much all that was needed to give them a bright new image, supplemented perhaps with a few new items for the wardrobe.

It starts to become a little easier to turn the difficulties of wig wearing into a 'positive' if it is seen as an opportunity rather than a deficiency. When you get a new wig, think about choosing a new item of snazzy clothing at the same time. Not only does this give an extra boost to making you feel good, but it can also deflect your own and everyone else's attention from your hair. Eventually, your friends will not be sure exactly what has changed each time they see you! A change of appearance can make you more interesting (not less) to a partner.

Having finally accepted that I may now have to live without my hair for the rest of my life, it has taken some time for me to lose the feelings of sadness and resentment, to get to know what kind of wig suits me best and in what type and style I feel at my most confident. Alongside this I have found a new lifestyle and new interests to help me restore my enjoyment of life, such life changes being something that most women in their middle years have to face anyway. Fortunately, I have been blessed with the tremendous support and understanding of my husband (but I know that not everyone is as fortunate in this respect). Even so it has been a long process of personal adjustment, research, learning and experimentation.

The advice and tips that I have outlined are from my own personal experience and are offered genuinely. Of course, in the normal way of things these days, I must add the disclaimer that I can accept no responsibility whatsoever for the outcome of applying any of my suggestions or for the following of any of my advice.

Every woman must find her own preferred way of handling her difficulties and make her own choices. Every set of individual circumstances will be different. However, I hope that my thoughts and advice will help others, especially new and longer term hair loss sufferers, and will give them the encouragement to stay focussed on working a way through and out of the daily difficulties. I also hope that those caring for hair loss sufferers will come to a better understanding of the condition's practicalities and how to manage them.

I still know when I am having a bad hair day, for even wigs do not always do *exactly* what they're told! I never thought I would say this, but after wearing a wig for so long they have become a natural part of me and I almost feel lost without one. Putting a wig on in the morning is just like putting on a wristwatch, earrings, contact lenses or spectacles. It gets to be routine.

It is so easy to experiment with styles, colours, lengths and cuts, short or curly, dark or light, and you do not have to wait for a bad style to grow out. If you get bored with one look, simply put on another one. With a little experience, effort and determination, you can look as good as you ever did.

The real bonus is that you can actually come to look even better than you did before. This is especially true for those more senior ladies, whose own hair would invariably become thinner and, perhaps because of this, less attractive over the years. Looking groomed and attractive, perhaps with a modern style (sometimes only possible with a wig) and age-sensible colour (difficult to achieve on naturally all white or grey hair), can seem to take years off a woman and make her feel really great. More importantly, feeling good from the inside can contribute to overall mental well-being and physical health.

If you find that you have to wear a wig for the rest of your life, do not be too downhearted for you may well end up having the best deal of all. As those around you complain more and more about their own natural hair, you can smile a little smile to your inner self. Unlike your friends, you can look just exactly the way you choose to look every day and every time of day. The advantages you have over those with their own hair will probably get better and better every year. The best thing is that the more years you wear a wig, the better you will get to look.

Be feminine because you are.

Feel good because you can.

Look great because you do.

And go out and be fantastic!

Some special sensitivities

The early days of discovering the hair loss problem

Anyone seeing the evidence or asking questions

Removing a wig to be medically-examined

Dealing with personal relationships

Windy days – they generate a feeling of great
insecurity, especially for full wig wearers

Breezy summer days – wearing a hood or hat
for security is not as acceptable as it is in winter

Going on open boats or walking to airplanes
and helicopters; hill walking or any place exposed
to adverse weather

Games or sports that involve energetic movements;
running; the chance of being jostled, pulled or hit

Bright sunshine and bright lights –
these can show up the artificial nature of wig fibres
or reveal a wig's construction

Wet weather – wetting a wig can expose its
structure; a real hair wig may be difficult to dry
and re-style

special sensitivities...

Getting the head wet on beaches or when swimming

Dogs that leap up and can cause nervousness and
disarray

Crowded, jostling places; shops and clubs

Babies and youngsters - they love to grab at hair or
play with hair strands; they will also be without tact
if they think something is 'wrong' or different

Smokers, fire and candles – not only will a wig
absorb the smoke smell but heat and fire is
potentially hazardous

Trying on clothes, especially in public, if they have to
be pulled over the head; using changing rooms can
be worrying and embarrassing

Putting on and then taking off a hat or hood

Fan ovens, grills, outdoor patio heaters - hot air can
damage a wig permanently

Talking about hair or hairdressers – it draws
unwanted attention to head hair

Jokes about baldness or wigs

Being touched on the head, or hugged

special sensitivities...

Being photographed or videoed; seeing an old picture with own hair, or being 'framed' wearing a former wig

Someone trying to help cover up something that has become exposed – then the sufferer feels really sure that the problem shows, even when the other person is only trying to help

Some advantages of wigs

Have a new colour and style - it's so easy!

Alternate your colours and styles in a single day

Change a colour to suit your mood and clothing

Get 'ready' effortlessly in the mornings

Be dressed quickly to go out at short notice

Have great fun choosing and trying out different looks

Your partner can enjoy your changes!

You can freshen up with a quick wig-switch

Banish greasy, dry or difficult hair days

No more inconvenient hairdresser appointments

No more potential haircut or style 'disasters'

On hot days - take wigs off to swim or cool off, wear a cooling pack underneath them or chill them in the 'fridge

No more thin or colourless patches as you get older

Be admired and envied

Index